PRAISE FOR THE AEROBOX® PROGRAM,
A FITNESS KNOCKOUT!

"A HIGH INTENSITY WORKOUT ALMOST ANYONE CAN DO. THIS REV-YOU-UP, RESULTS-ORIENTED EXERCISE PROGRAM STREAMLINES THE BODY, BUILDS UP ENDURANCE, AND INCREASES SPEED AND AGILITY LEVELS."

—Healthwatch

"PACKS AN AEROBIC PUNCH...THE ONLY REQUIREMENT IS THAT ONE NEEDS A STRONG DESIRE TO PUSH HIS OR HER BODY TO THE LIMIT. AEROBOX...is not simply a blend of aerobics and boxing. The prograrn focuses on basic boxing moves, different punches and footwork, calisthenics, and rope jumping."

—New York Newsday

"AEROBOX IS AN HOUR OF ASTONISHINGLY FAST PUNCHING EXERCISES and rope jumping."

—Newsweek

"A HARD-HITTING, NONCONTACT WORKOUT THAT TONES THE BODY BIG-TIME, AND ALSO INCREASES STAMINA, SPEED, AND AGILITY....A serious contender on the exercise scene."

—Toronto Sun

"HELPS RELIEVE MENTAL PRESSURE LIKE NO OTHER EXERCISE CAN...gives participants the cardiovascular conditioning they need...an all-encompassing workout."

—Metro Sports Magazine

"AEROBOX IS AEROBICS GONE HARD-CORE."

—British Elle

"IT'S A CARDIOVASCULAR WORKOUT AND AN EGO BOOST FOR MEN, AND WOMEN FEEL A SENSE OF POWER AFTER COMPLETING IT."

—Kacy Duke, aerobics director, Equinox fitness club

"MICHAEL OLAJIDÉ [JR.] AND HIS AEROBOX ARE PUTTING CONVENTIONAL EXERCISE AGAINST THE ROPES."

—French Glamour

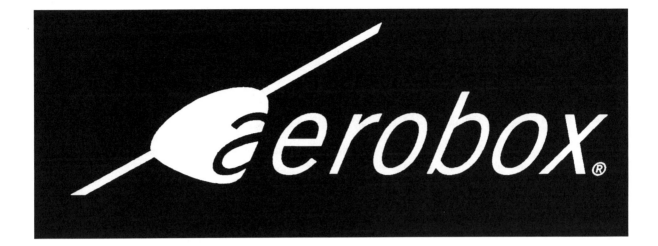

A
HIGH
PERFORMANCE
FITNESS
PROGRAM

■

MICHAEL
OLAJIDÉ, JR.

WITH PHIL BERGER

WARNER BOOKS

A Time Warner Company

Aerobox® is a registered trademark of Aerobox Athletic Enterprises, Inc.

Copyright ©1995 by Michael Olajidé, Jr., and Pheo Productions
All rights reserved.

Warner Books, Inc., 1271 Avenue of the Americas, New York, NY 10020

W A Time Warner Company

Printed in the United States of America
First Printing: August 1995
10 9 8 7 6 5 4 3 2 1

Library of Congress Cataloging-in-Publication Data

Olajidé, Michael.
    Aerobox : a high performance fitness program / Michael Olajidé,
Jr., with Phil Berger.
        p.   cm.
    Includes index.
    ISBN 0-446-67116-9 (pbk.)
    1. Physical fitness. 2. Aerobic exercises. 3. Boxing (Sport)
I. Title.
GV481.0346   1995
613.7'11—dc20   94-42162
                                                         CIP

Cover design by Julia Kushnirsky
Photography by Jesse Frohman
Book design by Giorgetta Bell McRee

*My efforts in this book are dedicated to
my family and friends. One and the same.*

ACKNOWLEDGMENTS

I would like to express my deep gratitude to all those who have been a positive influence in my life, both personally and professionally. First, and always, my parents: thank you mother and father. And my siblings: David, Sandra, Tracy, and Tokunbo. I love you.

I would also like to thank Michael P. DiRaimondo, Steve "America's Singing Poet" DePass, and Hector Roca, three wise and great teachers from whom I have learned so much. And then there is Dr. A. Alessandro Pireno, whose influence on my life has been so profound that I find it hard to find the words to express my thanks. For eight years he has not only seen me through physical, emotional, and financial upheavals, but has sustained me with his steady belief that life has good things in store for me. He gave to me generously and selflessly. Thank you, Doc, for being there. Thanks, too, to Dr. Pireno's wife, Barbara, and their entire family for whom I have the greatest love and respect.

I must also thank Saint Mary Ann Levesque, Rob Fernandez, and Beverly Bond for their time and efforts and for appearing in this book. Cool shutterbug Jesse Frohman, thanks for your artistry. And thank you Tom Casino. Surely Muhammad Ali would declare you "the greatest boxing photog of all time!" My deep gratitude, too, to Andrew "the visionary" Brucker whose creative eye put the stamp of approval on this book. (Be sure to catch Andrew's ending shot, "Boxing only.")

Thank you Leslie Schaenman. This project would have been a lot harder without your help. To my coauthor, Phil Berger, our spirited editor, Jamie Raab, and her colleagues at Warner Books, thanks so much for believing in Aerobox. I'm forever grateful to "fitness phenom" Kathy Smith, Russ Kamalski, and Joanne Feldman of BodyVision. Thank you for launching Aerobox. And, finally (I've always wanted to say this), a special SHOUT OUT to: Leslie Howes for the start of Aerobox; to the Errico family, owners of the Equinox Fitness Clubs N.Y.C., for the momentum; Teddy Singleton; Bob Gutkowski; Bobby Goodman; Angelo Dundee; Patricia Saracini and Benetton Sportsystem; my father's Kingsway Boxing Gym; Bruce Silverglade, owner of Gleason's Boxing Gym; George Wolfe; Oliver Mayer; Lord G; Moishe; Dingo; and Tyra.

Peace.

CONTENTS

INTRODUCTION: MICHAEL OLAJIDÉ, JR., ON AEROBOX   *xi*

PART ONE: THE BASICS OF AEROBOX   *1*
1   THE EXERCISE BLOCKS   *3*
2   PUNCHING   *7*
3   FOOTWORK/PUNCHING WHILE MOVING   *21*
4   SKIPPING ROPE   *29*
5   BODY TONING/ABDOMINALS   *39*
6   LIMBERING AND STRETCHING   *43*
7   FAMOUS LAST WORDS   *45*

PART TWO: THE AEROBOX WORKOUTS   *47*
8   MIND OVER MATTER   *49*
9   REALITY CHECK   *51*
10   HEAVY BREATHING   *53*
11   GETTING READY   *57*
12   THE BEGINNER'S WORKOUT   *61*
13   THE ADVANCED WORKOUT   *105*

PART THREE: THE AEROBOX COMPENDIUM   *137*
THE SUBJECT IS PARTNERS   *140*
THE TELEPHONE QUESTION   *142*
FATHER KNOWS BEST   *143*
WOMEN IN AEROBOX, PART I   *144*
WOMEN IN AEROBOX, PART II   *145*
SPOT TONING   *147*
GOOD PAIN, BAD PAIN   *149*
THE IMPORTANCE OF THE CLENCHED FIST   *150*
ANOTHER INJURY CONCERN   *150*
BURNOUT   *151*
OLAJIDÉ ON OLAJIDÉ   *152*
THAT EYE PATCH   *154*
AND FINALLY, YOUR AEROBOX TEST OF TESTS   *154*

GLOSSARY   *165*

INDEX   *167*

INTRODUCTION:
MICHAEL OLAJIDÉ, JR., ON AEROBOX

From 1981 until an eye injury forced me to retire in 1991, I was a professional boxer—a middleweight good enough to fight main events on national TV, to be ranked in the top ten by the sport's governing bodies, and twice to get world-title shots, including a prime-time bout against Thomas Hearns.

When I left boxing, with a record of 27-4 (19 knockouts), I continued to do a fighter's workout, but without the physical contact or bag punching that I'd done as a pro. My workout consisted of making all the moves of a fighter, but doing it now to a hard-driving beat.

In 1991, a New York City health club asked me to work one-on-one with its clientele, putting them through a boxing workout that would incorporate hand pads and the speed and heavy bags. I persuaded the club to let me try out the regimen that I had been developing, an aerobic format that was rooted in the intricate techniques and rhythmic movement of boxing.

Most people associate boxing with violence. And while boxing is a hard, brutal business, there is more to it than meets the eye. Think of Muhammad Ali, Sugar Ray Robinson, even Mike Tyson. Each had an original way of moving about the ring—the punches flowing off a beat that was as unique to each fighter as his thumbprint.

That movement—while stylized by the great fighters—has a common core. Boxing, like other sports, can be stripped to its basics. That is what Aerobox is about. I focus on the techniques of boxing, managing to work both upper and lower body while acquainting an individual with the disciplines of punching, footwork, and skipping rope in a noncontact format.

The notion of combining the rudiments of a fighter's discipline with the intensity of a cardiovascular workout was appealing, it turned out, to a lot of men and women. For every time I'd conduct a one-on-one Aerobox session, other people in the gym would watch in fascination and ask afterward if they could try it too. To my surprise, many of them were women. It didn't take long to see what the future held for Aerobox.

Aerobox is accessible to every level of athlete. The key is to work at the pace that suits your capacity. For the beginner, Aerobox can light the spark that begins a lifelong passion for fitness. For the experienced athlete, Aerobox is a perpetual challenge. While we may not spar or hit bags in Aerobox, believe me it's a demanding athletic workout—and not meant for the fainthearted.

Some of my earliest critics were fellow professional fighters, who felt I was exploiting my boxing past by creating a sissy's workout. Well, I don't hear that anymore. I've had professional fighters come to the health clubs at which I teach, thinking they're in for an easy time. And afterward they apologize, conceding that Aerobox is a great conditioning tool. Like the ex-world-champion middleweight who lasted only twenty-five minutes of what was to be an hour workout and was perspiring so extremely that we had to give him another T-shirt to go home in. Another ex-champion, World Boxing Organization middleweight king Doug DeWitt, had to take several rest breaks to last the session and later told me: "Geez, this workout gets it all."

That's typical. Athletes recognize that Aerobox is a stiff test for them. I worked two weeks in training camp with the New York Jets, who huffed, puffed, and groaned ... and afterward commended me for the hard work Aerobox provided them.

That challenge stirs the competitive juices of lay athletes too. It's amazing how quickly, in their enthusiasm, they catch on to the intricacies of Aerobox. In a matter of weeks, most of them go from bumblers on the skip rope to being very slick, and the same with all the boxing moves they need to master.

Aerobox is a workout that builds aerobic capacity while giving a sense of the movement of boxing. Guys love it because it's got the macho act of firing punches, and using the same bob and weave that we pros do to elude punches. So men who'd avoided aerobics in the past because it seemed too dance-oriented get the release they need.

Women love the workout for the intricacy of technique. In Aerobox, I teach how to stand, how to make a fist, the proper way to throw each and every punch—jab, right hand, left hook, uppercut. You do all this to music and you do it at a pace as intense as you can handle.

For women, it's also a way of getting acquainted with what seems an uncommonly violent sport, and coming away with an appreciation of the subtleties involved. And the funny thing is that women tend to take to the technical aspect of boxing more readily than the guys, who get their kicks out of unleashing energy through working the way a fighter does.

In Aerobox, besides moving and punching, we use the jump rope and push-ups, sit-ups, and stretching as well. Aerobox is a total body workout. It's varied and comprehensive. Whatever moves we make from a right-handed stance, we repeat as left-handers so that we build the total body.

Aerobox is hard work but not without its share of fun. I work in the Ali Shuffle, fancy skip-rope techniques, lots of stuff like that. Aerobox is also heavy on visualization. I ask my class to imagine the opponent in front of them as they move.

In this book, I walk you through the same arduous workout I give in the fitness studio, but in far more detail. You don't need to invest in expensive weight machines or join a high-priced health club. You can do Aerobox anywhere—in your home or, when you're traveling, in your hotel room. All you need is the book, a jump rope, and a willingness to work.

While Aerobox is geared for those who want the conditioning essence of boxing—get fit without getting hit—it also can serve as a training supplement for the myriad men and women who work out in fight gyms, hitting heavy bags and speed bags and sparring.

While I may not box for a living anymore, I still feel linked to the sport through Aerobox—and through the increasing number of people who are finding out what we fighters have known all along: boxing is one tough, demanding sport. And in the boxing-based format I conceived, it can keep you fit for life.

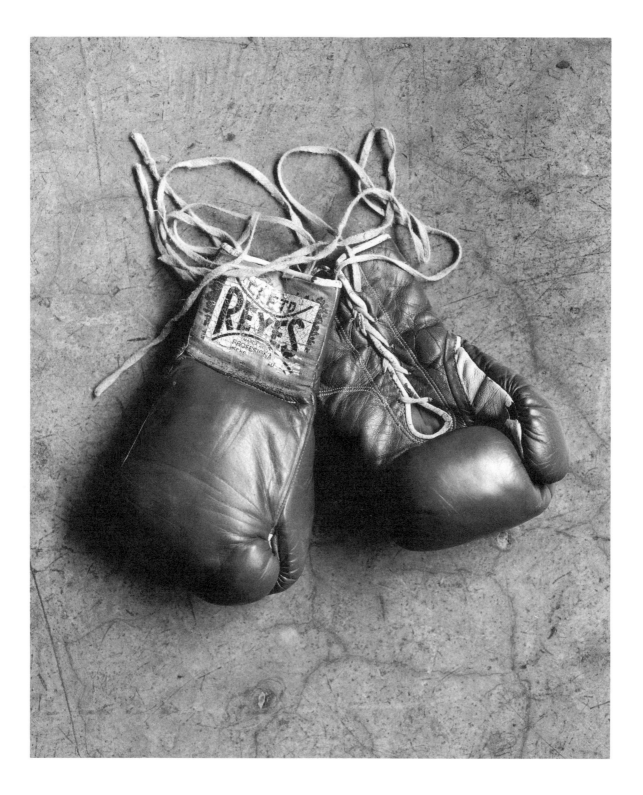

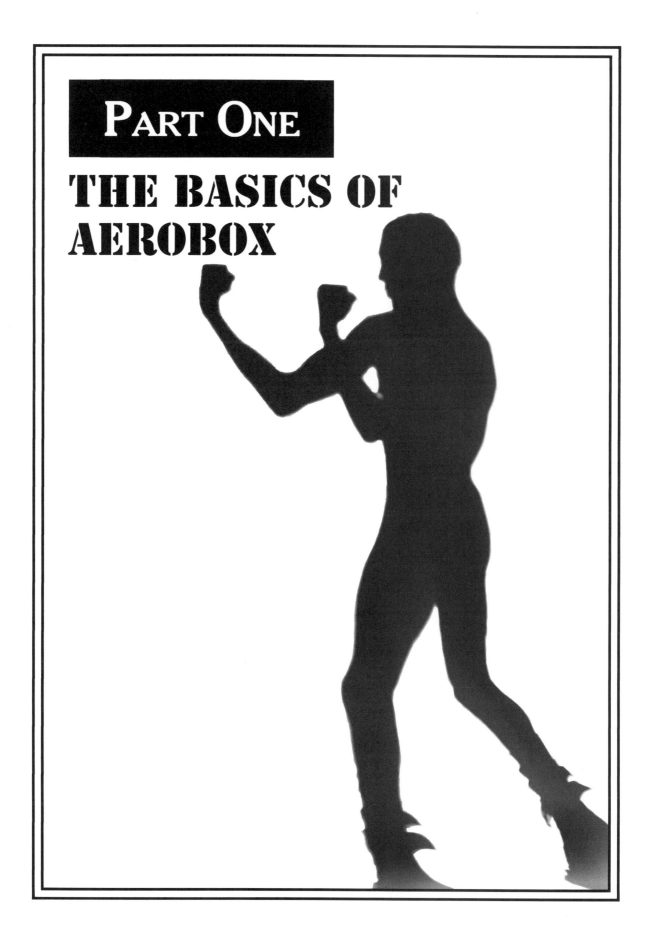

PART ONE

THE BASICS OF AEROBOX

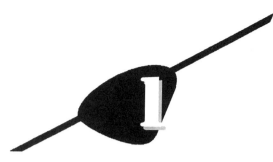

1

THE EXERCISE BLOCKS

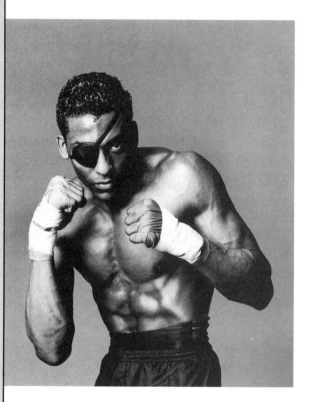

Like any worthwhile exercise regimen, Aerobox is a full-body workout.

While movement is at the heart of the workout, it is movement heightened by enough pinpoint exertions to tax the upper and lower body.

The pace—and intensity—of the workout will increase your aerobic capacity. But the demands on your limbs and torso will make you stronger if you are willing to do the work—an hour a day three times a week.

A word of caution, though. Don't expect to look and move like a veteran fighter in the blink of an eye. Rome wasn't built in a day, and no fighter ever was either. Including me.

As a youth growing up in Vancouver, British Columbia, and training under my father, I struggled, as everybody does, to master the fundamentals of my sport.

Eventually, I got to where most

of the techniques became instinctive. I was like a finely honed instrument when it came to administering my punches and eluding those of other men.

But the point here is: my skill level took time to develop . . . and so will yours. Don't be discouraged if you feel a bit awkward at first. Boxing is a sport of intricacies that are mastered by repetition, the slow but steady sharpening of muscle memory.

In Aerobox, it is not simply a matter of moving your feet, or simply a matter of throwing a punch. The objective is to be able to do both in harmony. And that's easier said than done.

Remember a few years back when comedians used to joke about President Gerald Ford lacking the dexterity to chew gum and walk at the same time? Well, the premise is pretty much the same here. It takes a bit of concentration, and practice, to move and throw a punch with competence.

On occasion in this book, I may use masculine pronouns like "he" and "his" to make a point. But rest assured that Aerobox is as much for women as it is for men.

Aerobox is comprised of seven exercise blocks—some fairly simple, some more intricate. A professional fighter's workout includes these same exercise blocks as well as regular sparring sessions. For those of you not conversant with the term, sparring sessions amount to the daily contact work for the fighter. He and his sparring partner wear protective headgear and box with gloves that are more heavily padded than they would be in a real match. By contrast, Aerobox is a noncontact format that concentrates more on the techniques involved in each exercise block and then blends them in an accelerated routine aimed at bringing you to your cardiovascular threshold.

The exercise blocks that make up your workload are:

1. Punching
2. Footwork
3. Punching while moving
4. Skipping rope
5. Body toning
6. Abdominal work
7. Limbering up and stretching

The exercise block is to Aerobox what the musical note is to the melody. The note, like the exercise block, may stand alone, but it is not until it is blended with other notes that the impact is of any consequence.

In practical terms, that means that you need to understand and then master all these facets of the Aerobox workout so that you can get the full benefit of your effort. Integrate the seven exercise blocks over an hour, as my classes do, and the result will be a workout that makes you feel good . . . and makes you fit.

Finally, a few words about how to approach this book.

What follows in Part One is a kind of big picture of Aerobox, analyzing its elements, with the occasional sidebar in which I expand on various facets of boxing as I experienced them during my professional career.

Pay particular attention to the more detailed material on how to punch and how to move when executing those punches. Absorb the technical descriptions and try them out in front of a mirror. You might want to do the same with your jump rope—a technique that, if you haven't ever done it, takes a little getting used to. A passing acquaintance with these exercise blocks will make the workouts seem far less alien when you get to them.

Part Two is all about those workouts—first some introductory remarks and then a step-by-step walk-through of the beginner's and advanced regimens. Each workout is accompanied by photos meant to make absolutely clear how to perform the various exercises that constitute Aerobox. I recommend you read through the text before actually doing your workouts. Familiarize yourself with what you will be doing so that when, finally, you strip down for action you won't be wasting time trying to comprehend just what it is you are to do.

Part Three is a compendium of Aerobox-related topics that includes a special elite workout for those who think they have the right stuff to do it.

That's what awaits you in these pages. But as with any new exercise program, I recommend that you consult with a physician before embarking on Aerobox. Once you've gotten medical clearance, and you begin doing the work, you're headed for a fit future.

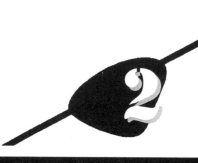

PUNCHING

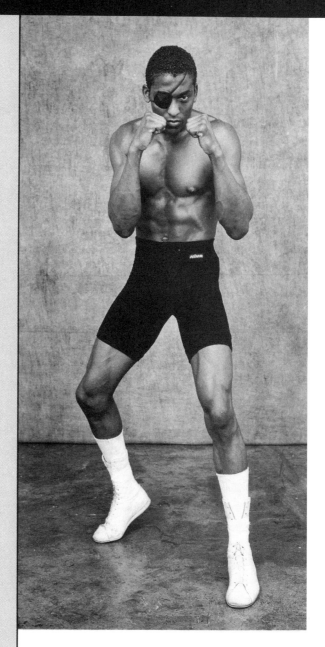

The Aerobox workout uses a fighter's punches as a kind of wind-up key to simple and then more intricate exertions.

At the beginning of the hour-long session, punches are thrown by the numbers, so to speak: slowly and with attention to proper form. This serves to ensure that the punches get delivered in a technically correct manner while the muscles involved get properly warmed up.

But first, let's be sure you've got your stance right.

What you want—assuming you're a right-hander—is to have your left foot forward, right foot back, and your knees slightly bent. Keep your weight centered and your body slightly tense so that punches will flow with force.

A fighter never presents a full target, so don't square up to your imaginary opponent. Your feet should be shoulder width apart, with your body at three-quarters profile to the foe. The toes of your left foot point forward, to twelve o'clock. Point the right foot to two o'clock. Your left shoulder is angled ahead of the right. Your chin is down.

Remember: do not place your right foot directly behind your left, as if you were walking a tightrope. The feet are apart and staggered back. This will give you mobility and balance.

The abdominal muscles should be flexed when punching, and your back should be straight. The shoulders are slightly hunched forward—think of a cobra ready to strike. Do not exaggerate this stance. Be subtle. But maintain that semitense state. In a fighter it makes his reflexes sharper and gives his every movement a force it would not otherwise have.

That tension in an athlete is a reflection of natural fear—and is the body's way of coping with it. Mike Tyson has talked openly of being lectured about fear, as a teenage prospect, by his mentor, Cus D'Amato.

Recalled Tyson: "I'd tell Cus after a fight, 'Cus, I was so scared.' 'It's natural,' he'd say. 'That's how come you're so good. When you're afraid, you're faster, you punch harder. It's just an aspect of what you do.'"

(For left-handers, when assuming your stance, just reverse the foot placement and, rather than fronting your opponent with your left side, lead with your right side at three-quarters profile.)

The objective is to have a stance that enables you to maintain equilibrium at all times.

Now for your hands. Put them in what we refer to as pyramid position—each hand to the side of the jaw so that your face is framed by those balled fists. Tilt the fists inward at the wrists and keep the chin between the hands. The fists should be about six inches in advance of your face and close to each other without touching. (See page 7.)

Why do we call this the pyramid position? Well, imagine extending the plane of your forearms and hands beyond their upraised position and the shape of those lines would surely be pyramidal.

When the hands are in pyramid position, not only do they afford a first line of defense, but from that angle they enable you to deliver a punch most efficiently.

In making a fist, you place the thumb outside the closed fingers and across the four middle phalanxes of your fingers. That's the area just below mid-finger and just above the segment that includes your nails.

Finally, your elbows. They hang a little wider, naturally, than your hands do. But consider them part of your defensive wall and keep them tight to your body. When your elbows are positioned like that, you can use them to obstruct and parry imaginary punches aimed at your stomach and ribs.

Now that your hands are raised and you've taken a secure stance, we are ready to learn the fighter's repertoire of punches.

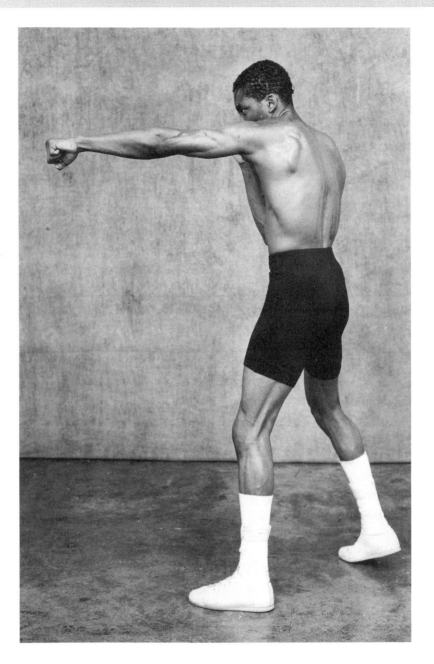

THE JAB
(muscles worked: deltoids, pectorals, triceps, biceps, trapezius)

Fighters use the jab in a variety of ways.

Typically, it is a punch that probes the opponent's defense, creating the openings for the heavier punches in a fighter's arsenal.

The jab is executed with the lead hand. Right-handed fighters throw the jab with their left. Southpaws use their right.

For most boxers, the jab is a punch off which a sequence of blows can be launched—"combinations" in the boxing vernacular. Those combinations are the assault weapons by which a fighter seeks to disassemble an opponent.

For the average fighter the jab is not regarded as a power punch. But there are men—like, say, Larry Holmes and George Foreman—whose jabs are heavy-handed: the punch can drive an opponent backward and, delivered in sufficient number, their cumulative force can numb the senses and produce swelling around the eyes and nose.

In January 1993, I saw a forty-three-year-old Foreman pound a young South African boxer named Pierre Coetzer with an unrelenting volley of jabs, round after round, that left Coetzer so bloody and defenseless that the referee was obliged to stop the fight by the eighth round.

When thrown in volume, a less energized jab can be an effective tool for disconcerting opponents, and keeping them so busy defending themselves that their chances of inflicting damage are diminished.

Whatever a fighter's intention, the jab is usually a prerequisite to success. For Aerobox, we throw the jab and other punches to tone the arms and give definition to the pectorals (pecs), deltoids, the trapezius muscles, the triceps, and the forearms.

How to deliver the jab?

The hands are in the pyramid position, the fists are closed. Elbows tight to the body. Thumbs outside the fingers, hands in front and at the sides of the chin. The left fist rotates so that it's parallel to the ground and face-high when extended . . . and the four head knuckles are pointed forward. (See page 9.) The fist is like the tip of an arrow. The elbow follows the hand's motion. You don't lift the elbow before uncorking the jab, for that serves to telegraph the punch.

When you jab, the punch comes off your lead foot, powered by your shoulder-area rotator cuff. Remember: you *do not* snap the elbow. The arm is extended 90 to 95 percent (so you don't hyperextend) and then it's pulled back to the set position without hesitation. As fast as the hand strikes forward, it must return. Out and back, out and back.

That speedy return to originating position is what enhances muscle definition, creating resistance that is similar to what you overcome when you curl a dumbbell. You always want to bring your jab back to set position. For women who are concerned about the excess flesh on the back of their arms, that triceps area gets maximum benefit (and tightening) when you complete the motion.

When shadow boxing or striking an inanimate object, make sure the knuckles of the index and middle fingers strike first. This is important because those fingers and the knuckles are the strongest part of the fist. Visualize making contact at face height.

The jab is often a probing maneuver, exploratory in intention. A fighter may use it to gauge the opponent's reactions and distance. But the double jab is more like an act of aggression—two rapid-fire jabs, usually thrown as a precursor to the power punch.

The technical distinction here is that when the initial jab is delivered, you retract it only halfway to set position so you can unleash the second jab quickly and with power.

In Aerobox, while the jab initially is thrown from the orthodox (right-hand) stance, participants then shift to the southpaw position so that both sides of the body are worked equally. This approach is applied to all the punches executed in Aerobox and is what gives this format its comprehensiveness.

To walk through the various punches—the jabs and the power blows—might make you technically proficient, but it will not tax your body unless you are executing the punches, and moving, at the brisk pace that Aerobox mandates.

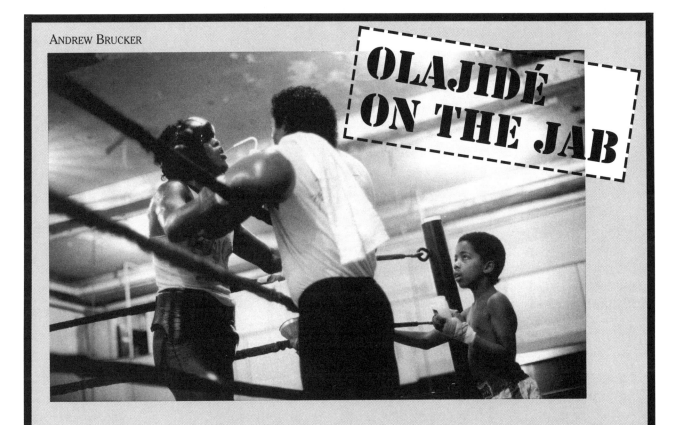

ANDREW BRUCKER

OLAJIDÉ ON THE JAB

I was fifteen years old when I first went into the Kingsway Boxing Gym in Vancouver. It was a ground-level, well-worn gym, with a sign that warned fighters not to spit on the floor.

My father owned the gym and, when he began training me, he told me right off that the jab was the most important weapon in boxing. And he made sure I got the point by standing me in front of a full-length mirror and having me throw the jab over and over again, hundreds of times, until I became sore because of the repetitiveness of the punch, pumping it out and back, out and back.

There were times I stood in front of the mirror for up to half an hour and did nothing but practice the jab. It was hardly glamorous work but it helped build my foundation as a fighter. I understood that and did the work without complaint. (At least I didn't complain as much as some others.) But lots of guys I started with couldn't see past the tedium and, taking the short-term view, gave up on the sport. It was a kind of litmus test for how serious you were. I was serious and would work endlessly to refine the jab. My arm would feel heavy, but over a period of time I built a resistance to fatigue. I was able to do it longer and faster.

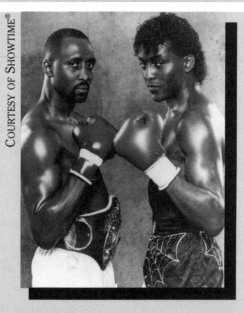

COURTESY OF SHOWTIME®

I developed a jab and, because I used it so much, the latissimus muscle on my left side became more pronounced than what I had on my right side.

I've seen some very potent jabs—and experienced a few. Like Thomas Hearns's. His jab was unique. Hearns is a tall, lean guy, who resists the orthodox approach by carrying his hands low—kind of like gunfighter-arrogant. But because of that, when he jabbed, it didn't come from where you expected. It started out of your field of vision almost, and came shooting up from his beltline. A very quick punch. Velocity that compounded the power. It reminded me of the way the knights in medieval times thrust their lances. The more speed generated, the more power it delivered.

Guys like Hearns—the jab is a stinging punch. Other guys have thudding jabs. I'm thinking of Foreman and Sonny Liston. Their jabs are not particularly quick, but it's like getting clubbed with a telephone pole. When that fist hits your head, it rocks the brain. You watch Foreman jab. It's like he's punching through the target. He has these immense arms and that jab is like a battering ram the way he throws it.

Holmes's jab was not from a set position. He came up with the jab. And boom—the right hand followed a split second later. That left-right is a very basic combination in boxing. When you hear somebody refer to "the old one-two," that's what they're talking about: the jab followed by a right hand thrown with, as Tyson liked to say, "bad intentions." Holmes did very well over the years with the one-two, and the jab was what made it particularly effective. He got attention with that jab. Bing bing bing—he put it in your face and then the right would come like a rifle shot, sneaking in there just behind the jab.

Most of the guys I've mentioned—Hearns, Holmes, Foreman—had long arms. And it's logical that a guy who has some reach, as they say, would have an edge at landing his jab. But there are short-armed guys who knew how to get their jabs across.

Roberto Duran was one of them. He had short arms, but he was a lot more clever than people gave him credit for. He'd time his move. When you threw your jab, he'd bend to the right and in the same motion shoot his jab, taking advantage of your momentum. Practically walking you into his jab. It was a little like an ambush. Very clever.

POWER PUNCHES

While the jab is an important weapon for a fighter, you do not put your body into it the way you do with your power punches—straight rights (or lefts), hooks, and uppercuts.

The difference is that the jab is powered by the muscles of the shoulder region, and the power punch comes off the back foot, involving the synchronized movement of your whole body.

COURTESY OF SHOWTIME®

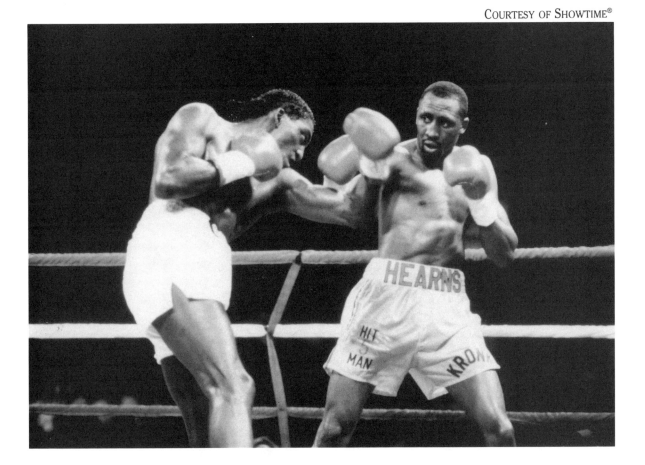

When you throw a punch off the back foot, you are transferring weight from the back foot forward by rotating your hips and shoulders. It's not unlike how a baseball player generates power when swinging at a pitch or a tennis player gets velocity on the forehand. That torque, in baseball, tennis, or boxing, is the source of an individual's power.

It is more fatiguing to throw power punches than just to jab. That's why most fighters limit the volume of hooks, uppercuts, and straight right hands (straight lefts if they're southpaws). No fighter wants to grow so exhausted he's susceptible to getting hit.

Aerobox takes the opposite approach—building up to rapid-fire combinations that work you to the max. Since nobody is going to hit you when you slow down, your pain is physical gain . . . with no bruises to show for it.

That gain is consistent with Aerobox's intent—to tax the entire body. With power punches you use your legs and turn your torso. The straight right (or left) requires you to rotate your upper body and use the rotator cuff. The uppercut stresses the obliques and lats. The hook, with its more insistent torque, demands more of the abs.

THE STRAIGHT RIGHT HAND
(muscles worked: abdominals, trapezius, latissimus dorsi, pectorals, and upper back)

In the one-two combination, the jab goes out first, diverting an opponent's attention, and/or lowering his guard, so that the straight right hand that follows can land like a wrecking ball against an unprotected face.

The thought of that may make you squeamish, but when a fighter lands that right unimpeded and knocks another man off his feet, invariably it is a moment that incites the crowd.

Okay. Here's how to deliver your power right. (Note: for a left-hander just reverse things.)

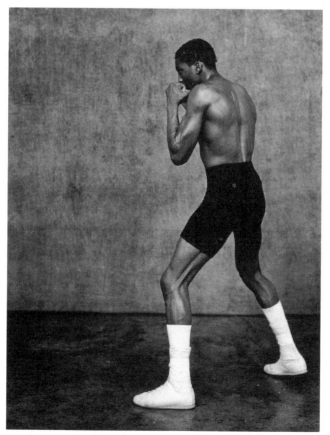

Assume your stance—weight evenly distributed, hands in the pyramid position. Shoulders rolled forward. Chin down. The right hand comes out from the cheek. As you unleash it, twist your body as though you're pushing open a big heavy door, your shoulders and hips rotating. Your right side will swing forward, as your left side swivels back.

Your feet grip the ground, your abdominal muscles (abs) are tight. Punching is a whole-body experience. Some movements are subtle, others not. Let your legs be the driving force. And breathe naturally.

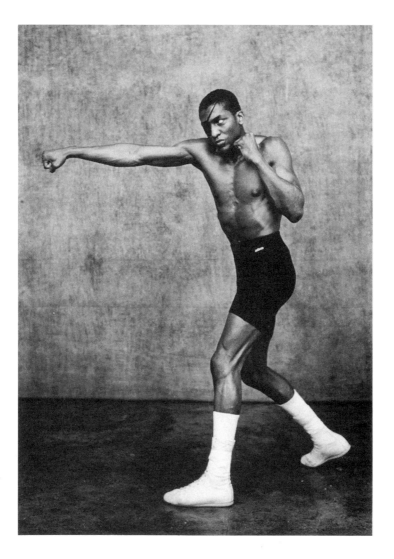

If the abs are tight and you rotate your torso, you are using your whole body in synchronization. Without that torque, there's no power generated.

When you deliver the blow, make sure the bottom of your fist is parallel to the ground. Drive the punch to where you visualize your target. Don't overextend the punch. Remember: keep the elbows tight to the body when not punching, and do not flap them like wings when letting the punch go.

Once the punch is delivered, retract your right hand and return to set position.

THE HOOK
(muscles worked: biceps, obliques, and upper back)

For a right-handed fighter, the left hook is a more complex punch. It is akin to the forehand in tennis—a learned stroke rather than the natural motion of a backhand one.

Yet some fighters throw a left hook as though it was their birthright. Former heavyweight champion Smokin' Joe Frazier could whale that left—remember the left that knocked Muhammad Ali down in their first fight, at Madison Square Garden in 1971. More recently, Julio César Chávez has proven expert at disturbing rib cages and abdomens with his left hook.

Guys like these make the punch look easy. But it's not easy. In fact, for newcomers I break the punch down into segments.

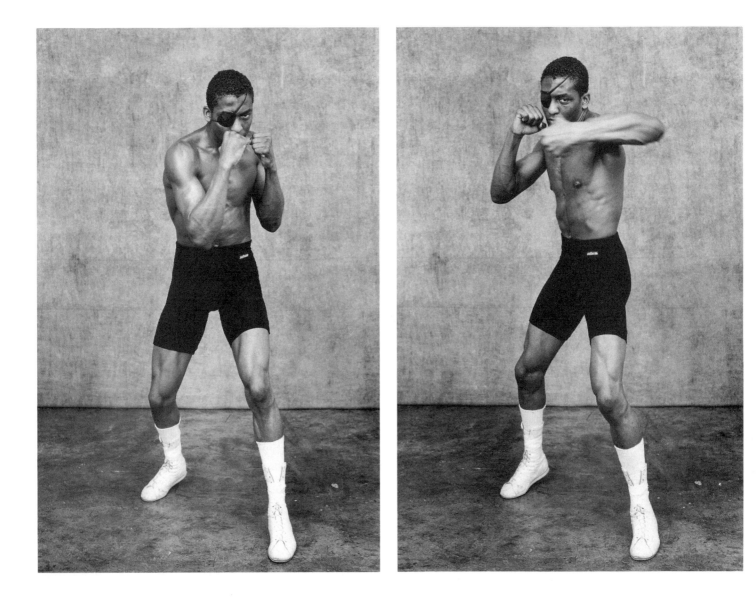

Consider the arm movement first. With your elbow shoulder high, the left hand swings outward and across the body, cutting a curving line that stops, say, eighteen to twenty-four inches out in front of you, face-high. Visualize impact occurring slightly past your nose. Don't let the punch go soaring beyond that point. At that moment, your palm should be facing you, not facing down. Do this movement without twisting your body. Just concentrate on the arc of the punch. Do it slowly once. Then do it slowly sixteen times.

Be careful not to swing the elbow back for a head start. It's a common mistake for beginners and leads to a punch that's more like a slap. The hook is driven from the shoulder. Your elbow is as high as the fist at the imaginary point of contact.

Now let's get the motion that accompanies the punch. With your elbows tight to your body, swing your left shoulder back slightly, as though cocking it. Then rotate that shoulder to the right, keeping your abs tight. This uncocking movement is the torque that gives the punch its power. As you rotate, your feet grip the ground, your knees are slightly bent. Again, you breathe naturally.

Practice rotating from the shoulders without incorporating the punch. Do the movement slowly, and repeat it sixteen times. Your shoulders should be rolled forward as you turn your body. Your legs have to supply some of the torque too.

In the final stage, we put both elements—the punch and the torque—together. As the body begins its torque, the arm swings up and out, in synch with the body's twisting. When the punch is executed, retract the fist along the same line, bringing the hand back to set position while slightly rotating the upper body.

THE UPPERCUT
(muscles worked: latissimus dorsi, obliques, trapezius, and biceps)

The uppercut is a blow driven upward into the opponent . . . in what, loosely speaking, is an underhanded motion. The same sort of motion you'd use when gripping the bottom of a window in your palm and pushing it up.

An uppercut is usually thrown at close quarters, and more often than not it is calculated to catch a fighter who works out of a crouch and relentlessly bores in.

An uppercut can be thrown with either hand, by a right-handed or left-handed fighter. For the purposes of our discussion, assume a right-handed fighter is delivering the uppercut with his right hand.

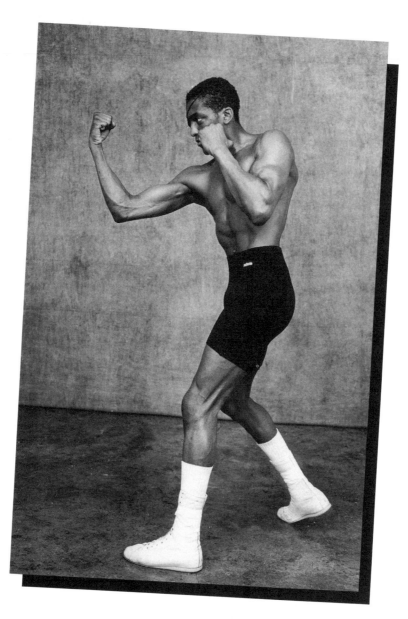

With your hands in set position, your front foot pointing at the opponent, you want to rotate the fist up and the shoulder out. The punch is stopped at face level, with the palm of your hand facing you, and ideally the opponent's jaw being the imagined contact point. Never let the uppercut soar over your head and shoulders. Once the punch is delivered, rotate the shoulder back and bring the hand to set position, never letting the elbow swing behind the body on the return of the punch.

Remember: this is a punch that works best at close quarters. When executed at long range, a fighter has a tendency to reach for his opponent, leaving himself wide open.

Back in October 1990, that is what the then-heavyweight champion, James (Buster) Douglas, did when he fought Evander Holyfield. From long range, he let fly a right uppercut that missed badly, exposing his jaw. Holyfield rocked back on his right foot, then drove a right hand from his shoulder, hitting Douglas on the jaw and knocking him out to win the heavyweight title.

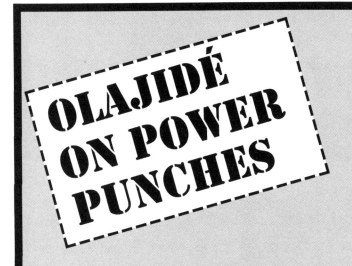

OLAJIDÉ ON POWER PUNCHES

You see a lot of fighters with Muscle Beach bodies who don't punch with real power. It's because they lack coordination. Their weight lifting diminishes their punching capabilities. The muscles in their shoulders and arms are locked to their torso. They don't have the flex, the ability to generate velocity.

That's the thing about hard punchers. They come in all shapes and sizes. Long spindly guys like Thomas Hearns and Bob Foster could hit like hell. And big-boned, hamfisted guys like George Foreman and Sonny Liston hammered guys into submission. Tyson had big, powerful thighs that, it seemed, lent his punches their torque.

But, for the most part, it's a mystery why certain guys have power and others don't. By that I mean you look at body types and they tell you nothing. Not until you see how a guy moves do you get an inkling about whether he can punch with power.

In Vancouver, when I was developing as a fighter, I used to hit a sandbag—a really hard sandbag. We called it our "power bag." It was supposed to develop your punching power. Who knows? Maybe it did. As a puncher, I was not in the same class as the Foremans and Tysons, but I was able to hurt strong, capable opponents just the same, knocking down Iran (The Blade) Barkley and staggering Thomas Hearns, both of whom were world champions. Sometimes, all it takes is timing—catching a guy when he doesn't expect the punch.

My theory is a lot of a fighter's punching power comes from his back. I believe that pull-ups, with a wide grip, can give you a lot of power, and are particularly good for skinny guys. Pull-ups tend to give you that V body and build up your lats. I say skinny guys with V backs are more likely to be heavy punchers.

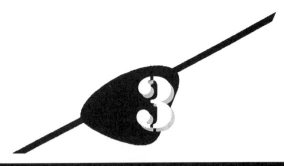

FOOTWORK / PUNCHING WHILE MOVING

*(muscles worked: those utilized in punches
and the gluteus maximus, quadriceps, and calves)*

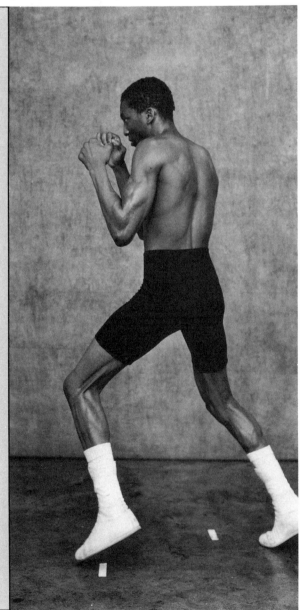

The fighter Willie Pep was before my time, but there's a story about him that will give you a sense of the artistry behind the way a boxer moves about the ring.

The story told to me by boxing writers is that Pep, a world-champion featherweight (126-pound limit) in the 1940s, once boasted that he would decisively win a round on the judges' scorecards without so much as throwing a punch. How? By moving so smartly—using feints and footwork to make the other man miss—that his dominance would be clear enough that he would not need to throw a punch.

And according to those newsmen who covered him, Pep made good on his boast, winning a round in which he never threw a punch but ended up making his opponent look ludicrous for trying to hit him. The opponent's punches soared wide of the target and, as Pep pivoted here and feinted there, he had the other man stumbling about like an amateur.

Now I'm not going to promise you that Aerobox will make you as slick as Willie Pep. But for sure you will understand how a fighter moves and what his objectives are when he negotiates the ring. Not to mention that your agility and balance will improve ... and your calves, thighs, and glutes will become more defined.

When I took up boxing, I was taught the stance and the jab, and then given the basics of movement. There were three guiding principles that I was expected to retain about traversing a boxing ring: One, always stay balanced. Two, whether moving forward or back, one foot follows the other and never do your feet come together. Three, as you advance, always come to the set position.

With those cardinal rules in mind, we can work through the most basic of boxing movements. Out of your stance, move your lead foot forward six inches, then advance your trail foot six inches. Come to the set position. Reverse the order as you move backward.

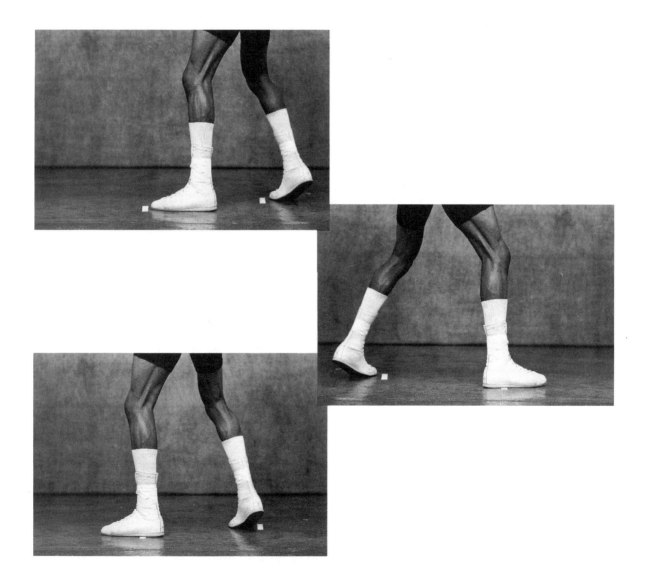

To move laterally, it's the same model. To slide laterally to the right, you step with your right foot first and your left foot follows. Reverse the order as you move laterally to the left.

Once you have the rudiments of movement—pretty simple stuff, really, if you've had even a little experience boxing—you're ready to throw the jab as you step.

When I'm conducting an Aerobox class, I talk the participants through their first efforts at combining movement and punches like this: "Okay, step forward and, as you do, the jab begins its forward movement. Now the hand returns to set position, just before you bring your rear foot forward so that you're in start position."

The more intricate side of footwork has to do with "slipping punches"—boxing jargon for the tutored way in which fighters duck a blow. These movements work the quadriceps and the gluteus maximus, aka the quads and glutes . . . and they enhance coordination at a low- to medium-impact range. Talking you through it, it goes like this:

"You're in the set position. The bend comes from the knees. The mistake a lot of people make is to bend their back and do a sweeping motion. Bending from the knee is key. Once you bend, you roll your body to the left and, as you straighten up, you bend at the knees again and roll your body to the right. It's a sweeping U or V motion. Got it?"

V-SLIP

"Okay. Visualize that punch aaannd . . . come under . . . under . . . and under. Always keeping that eye on the opponent. And never letting the knees surpass the edge of the toes. Under . . . and to the side. Under . . . and to the side."

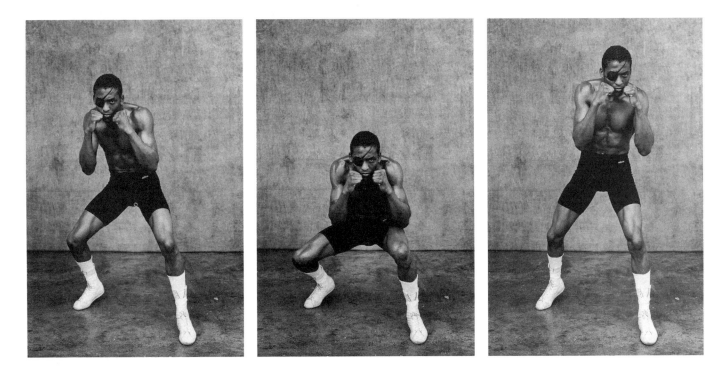

LATERAL SLIP

There is another form of slipping punches. In this maneuver, the feet remain in place and you flex the upper torso sideways—a quick shift that executed smartly will elude the punch and, for fitness' sake, will work your abs and your side muscles, the obliques.

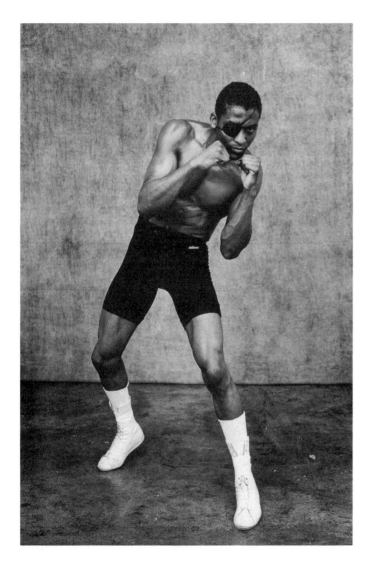

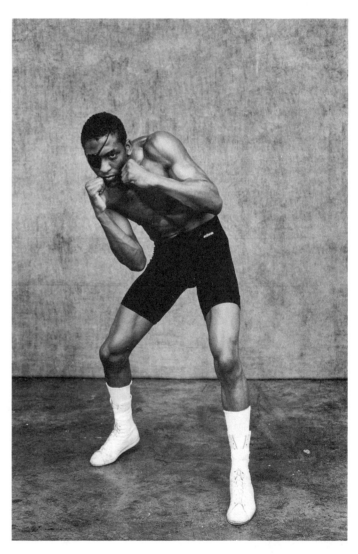

ALI LEAN

Ali was a master at twisting away or, as it's called, "riding a punch." He would lean back and to the left, twisting or turning from his waist, and his head would tilt in that direction too. He would never, however, lose sight of the man in front of him.

That's important for you to remember when you are slipping punches in the more conventional way. I've mentioned that the bend comes from the knees and not the back. The mistake that occurs when you bend from the back is more often than not you end up looking at the ground rather than at the opponent.

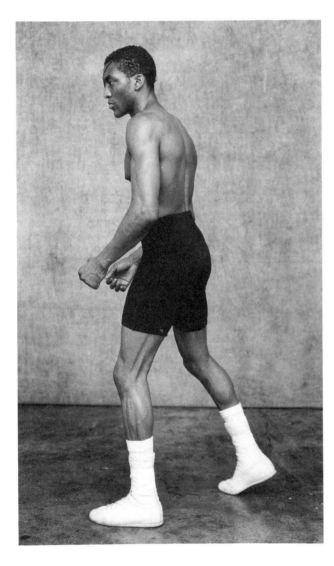

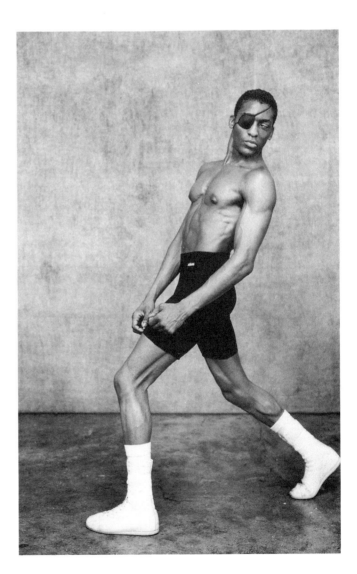

Ali aside—he was one of a kind—most fighters who are adept at evading punches bend from their knees. It's much more efficient using the knees . . . and not as fatiguing. In fact, when fighters who use their knees for slipping punches resort to using their back it's usually a clear sign that they are fatigued.

The purpose of slipping is not only to avoid being hit but to be in position then to counter your opponent. And in the progression of movements in the Aerobox repertoire, that is what you do next—slipping the punch and completing the movement by throwing a counterpunch of your own.

Beginners tend not to complete the slip move in their haste to unload that counterpunch. Don't hurry yourself. Finish slipping the punch before delivering your counter.

This is what elevates Aerobox into a heart-accelerating workout and makes it that rare experience of fun in a martial arts format. At its most intense, Aerobox demands that the participant move rapidly through assorted boxing arabesques—here firing punches in quick succession while moving forward, or backward, there slipping punches and countering. The succession of movements becomes a cumulative physical burden, taxing upper and lower body.

To reiterate: in the beginning, these movements may feel alien to you. Don't worry. Repetition will smooth out the rough edges. You may want to work in front of a mirror—a full-length mirror is best. There is nothing quite like watching yourself to gain a sense of the proper form.

For me, after a while proper form became second-nature. I did not need a mirror. Part of my mind would detach and become a sort of watchman, keenly aware of the nuances of movement. If, say, I was carrying my left hand too low, that vigilant "other" would sense it immediately and relay the message to the active self.

In time that will happen to you. Part of you will step aside and evaluate . . . and your technique and muscle memory will become refined.

Among professionals—and for you—that ability to be oblivious to everything but what you're doing is crucial. With concentration comes progress.

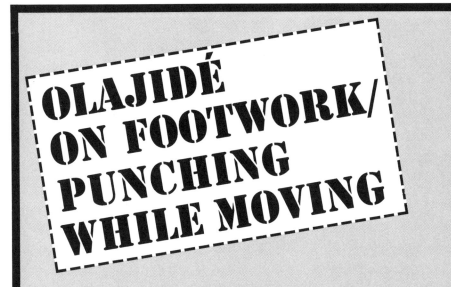

OLAJIDÉ ON FOOTWORK/ PUNCHING WHILE MOVING

Aerobox teaches a conventional style to keep confusion to a minimum—and to maximize conditioning benefits.

Aerobox is rooted in proper form, and adheres closely to the the style I used when I was fighting professionally. Sportswriters called me "The Silk," because of the smooth, technically clean lines of that style. Not that I was a fancy-dan. The flourishes were more cosmetic—tasseled laces and stylish robes and trunks. But the ring style was rooted in fundamentals passed down from generation to generation. Classic stuff.

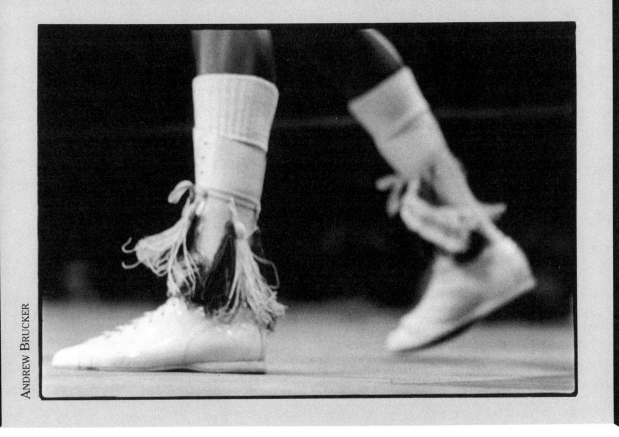

ANDREW BRUCKER

Yet in real life, some fighters move in ways that deviate from the orthodox approach It's not that they're willful about ignoring fundamentals. It's a matter of adapting tech-niques best suited to the particular dimensions of the fighter.

We look at dancers like Fred Astaire or Gregory Hines and we regard them as graceful Yet we're more reluctant to view a fighter who's extremely aggressive as having grace or finesse. When those ultra-aggressive fighters lack the sleek dimensions of an Astaire or Sugar Ray Robinson, they tend to be viewed as mere brutes and their artistry ignored.

By my view, though, it's a kind of snobbism to dismiss them that way. For instance, there are short-armed fighters like, say, Joe Frazier and Mike Tyson who developed the ability to get into position to deliver punches by clever moves honed hour after hour in the gym.

When the five-foot-eleven Frazier fought Ali, he was at a size disadvantage. The six-foot-three Ali had the height, and the reach, to keep him at long range, where he could outbox him. For Frazier to be effective, he needed to fight at close quarters. To get past Ali's piston jab, Frazier used exceptional foot and head movement.

Tyson was unique that way too. The popular notion was that he was a savage brawler, whose aggression and punch constituted all the assets he had. But in the early part of his career, up to when he knocked out Michael Spinks in ninety-one seconds in June 1988, Tyson was not only a devastating puncher but was remarkably elusive for a fighter who was so full-tilt aggressive.

It was no accident either that other fighters couldn't hit him. There was real art in the way he moved his head from side to side while in a crouch and, with the quickness of his feet, closed the distance between the opponent and him. His footwork and feints were so precise that he rarely got hit in spite of his seemingly reckless rushes forward.

Yet his life became more crazed after the Spinks fight. Some would say Tyson's concentration on technique slackened—that he got sloppy. To his critics, this seemed a reflection of his loss of interest in and concentration on his business. They pointed out that he abandoned the crouch and the tic-toc head movement to stand more erect and move forward without camouflaging his intentions. And they wrote that in abandon-ing technique he suddenly began getting hit. Cause and effect, they said. Following his first fight after Spinks, against Frank Bruno in February 1989, he was criticized for getting hit more times that night than he had in thirty-odd fights until then. Many of his critics felt it had less to do with Bruno—a strong but not especially gifted boxer—than with Tyson's sloppiness, disinterest, what-have-you. For them, it was no shock when Buster Douglas knocked him out a year later, in February 1990.

I never had to fight Tyson, thank God. But I can imagine how it must have been when he was coming up. All that head movement and elusiveness can get an opponent very tense. You don't know what he's going to do next ... or where the punch is coming from. If you want to punch him, you have to guess where he's going to be ... and think real hard about the punch he's going to respond with. Not easy. A lot of fighters were not up to the challenge.

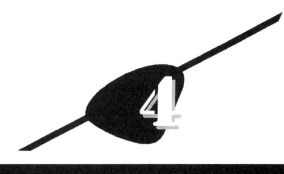

SKIPPING ROPE

(muscles worked: forearms, trapezius, thighs, calves, soleus, deltoids, pectorals, the muscles of your feet, and your cardiovascular system)

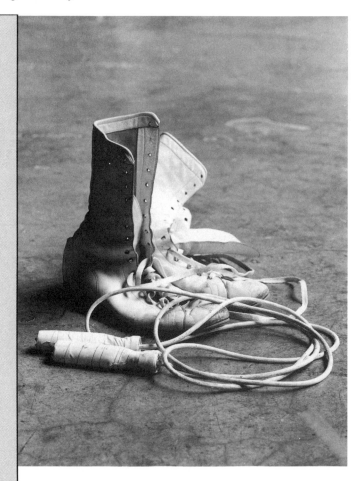

The clackety-clack of the rope against the floor has always been a familiar sound around the boxing gym.

Fighters use the rope for timing and conditioning. Most civilians marvel at the nonchalant way they whirl the rope and deftly jump over it.

To a boxing novice, it seems a marvelous stunt, like the trick shuffling of a deck of cards. But skipping rope—however effortless it may seem when a professional boxer does it—is demanding work. That makes it a hellacious fitness tool for the layman.

A word about that rope. A basic leather or plastic rope with ball-bearing handles costs twelve to fifteen dollars, and is just fine for what we do in Aerobox.

As with the punches and footwork you've learned, there are details of proper form to master. To begin with, you need to get comfortable with the rope, making sure that the length is right for your particular dimensions.

Here's how you do that. Grip the handles of the rope with both hands and then step on the rope, feet together. The arches of your feet should be over the rope. Your hands are palms up. You're standing there like a waiter holding a serving tray, arms perpendicular to your body.

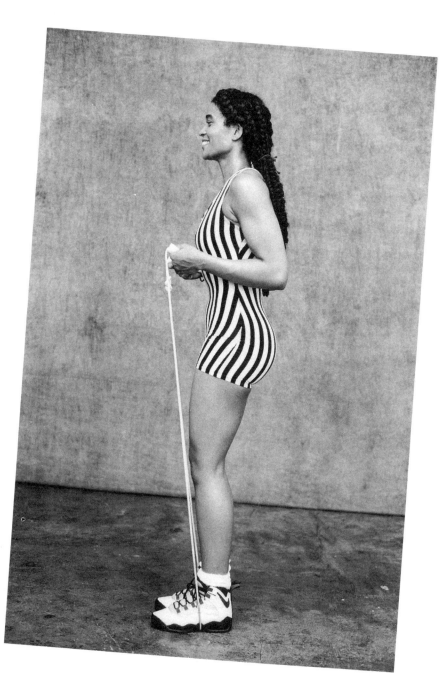

When you tug at the rope, it should come no higher than your solar plexus. If the rope is too long, do a simple slip knot close to the handle, and then measure it again. If the rope is still too long, put a knot on the other side. Your objective is to fashion a rope that doesn't have too much drag.

If, when you step on your rope, you discover the rope is too short, the answer is simple: buy another rope. Why's a short rope a problem? Because people tend to jump higher than they really need to with a short rope. If you jump too high, you can end up damaging your knees, feet, and shins from the pounding.

Once the rope is suited to your particular dimensions, it's time to get familiar with it. In Aerobox, we do that by standing in place and, with each hand gripping one of the handles, swinging the rope side to side.

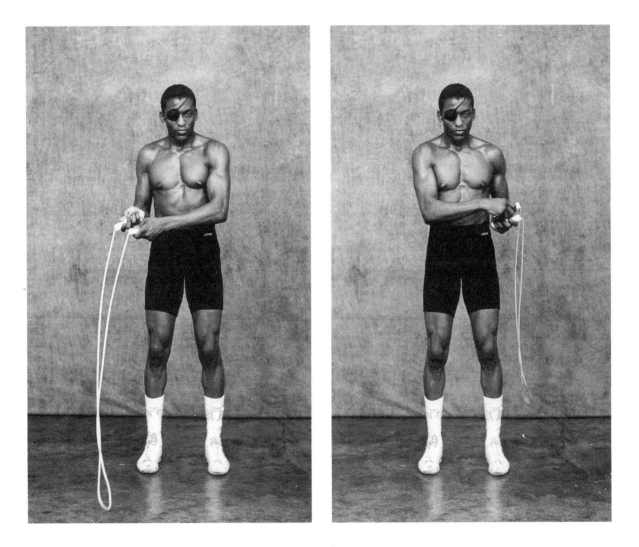

With your left hand on top and leading, you roll your wrists to the right, then roll them to the left. Your hands may come close to each other and maybe even touch. But never let them cross over each other. Your objective as you roll your wrists is to create a figure eight. When done correctly, the rope makes an X in front of you . . . and loops at the side—the portrait of that eight.

When you can move the rope side to side easily, it means you're comfortable enough with it to start jumping.

A few words first about common mistakes to avoid. The tendency among beginners is to jump too high. Or, as you jump, to kick your heels back toward your buttocks—an excess called jackknifing. Both of these approaches leave you susceptible to injury. What you're aiming for is a more casual, soft-shoe approach—something quick yet smooth. Semitense.

To start, your hands—gripping the rope handles—should be in front of your body, elbows close to the waist. You turn the rope from waist level, with your wrists rotating forward. The rope goes forward. It's an economical motion, as is your jump—no more than an inch and a half off the ground. One revolution per jump, with the wrists (and not the arms) powering the rope.

When you jump, push from the ball of your foot, with the heel leaving the ground before the toes do. The knees stay slightly bent, acting as shock absorbers.

Remember: it's with minimal movement that you get maximum benefits from the rope.

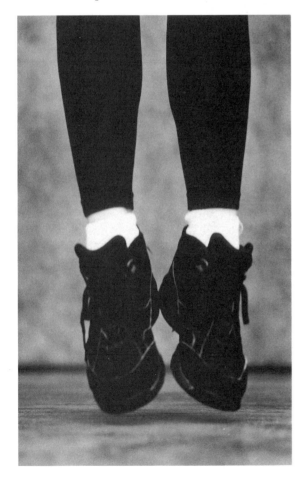

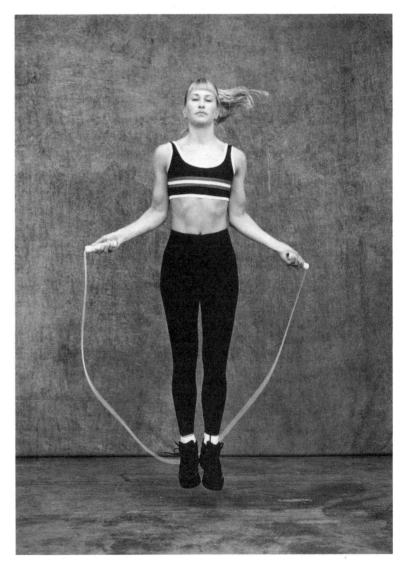

Once you're capable of sustaining thirty to sixty seconds of nonchalant rope jumping, you're going to aspire, inevitably, to the flashy maneuver called "crossing the rope."

That's when, amidst the whir of the rope turning, you flick your wrists at one another—the so-called crossing of the rope—and create a loop big enough for you to jump through.

Here's how you do it.

When you flick your wrists, your hands pass over each other and the loop materializes. The hands have to remain low. If you raise them, in anticipation of the move, you'll shorten your rope and screw up the maneuver.

When you cross the rope correctly, you will keep to the rhythm that preceded the maneuver. That means you're not changing your jumping pattern. You're merely shifting your hands. Do it that seamlessly and you're bound to draw admiring oooo's from friends and family. Which is half the fun of learning how to cross the rope. That ooooo.

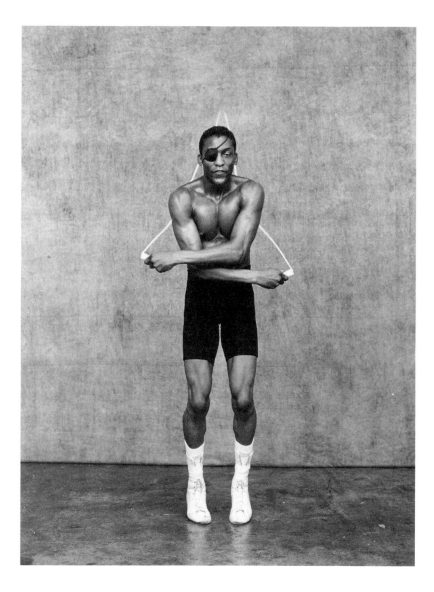

Skipping rope is repetitive and, without varying the routine, can become tedious. Aerobox starts with the basic pattern—two feet together, one revolution of the rope per jump—but it incorporates variations like crossovers with the rope and trickier footwork that gives you the feeling of being a skip-roping wizard.

For instance, you can do sideways jumps, feet together, that mimic the slalom effect of downhill skiing. It's great for the lateral muscles of the thighs . . . and the glutes.

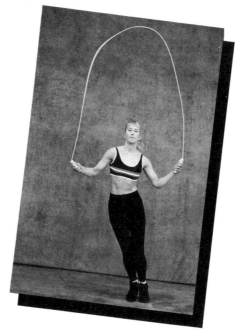

You can do the Ali Shuffle as the rope revolves, shuffling your feet back and forth rather than simply jumping. The timing is trickier, but not so difficult that it can't be accomplished with a bit of practice.

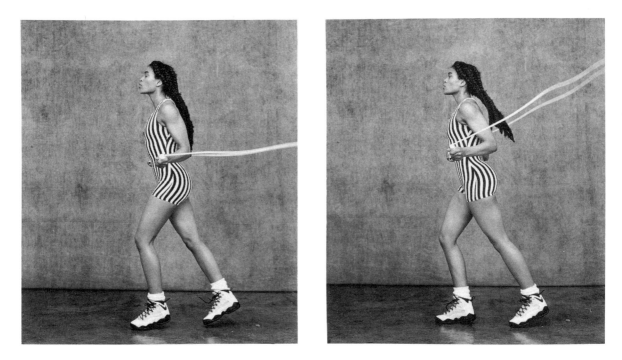

You can do a kind of Irish jig ("heel, toe, raise the foot to the back, bring it forward and across the knee") or running in place that mimics the rubber-tire drill that football players do (see page 36).

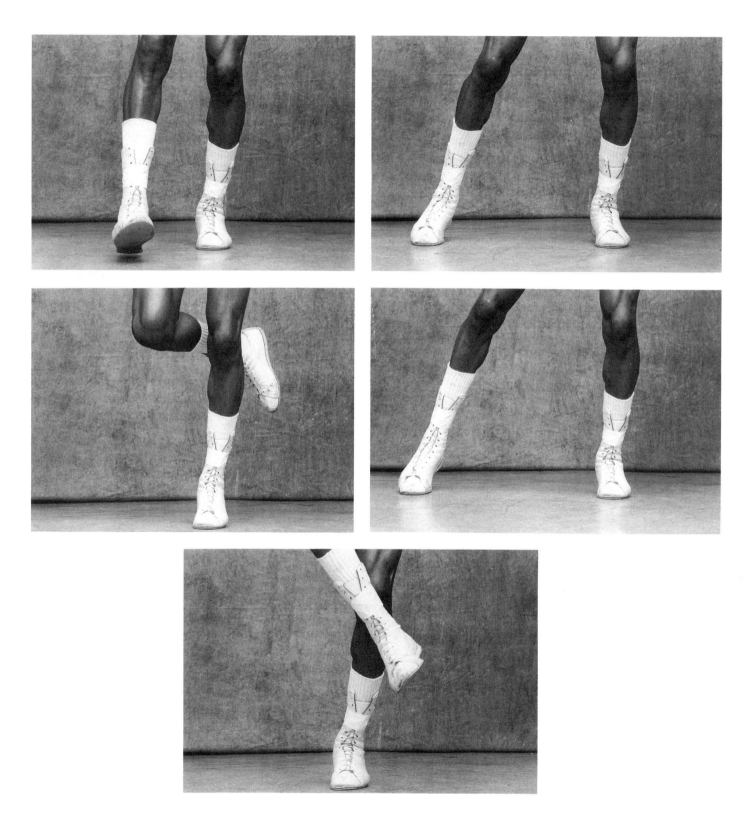

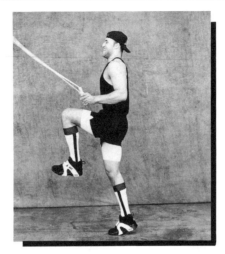

To take yourself to the aerobic threshold, you do a double jump. One magnified jump, with two rotations of the rope, as fast as you can. To execute this correctly, your body needs to be slightly rigid, with the tension centered at the rotating wrists. The jump is twice as high as your normal jump. This variation is the rope equivalent of wind sprints.

The rope provides enough cardiovascular intensity to satisfy the most demanding athletes. While it works the calves, quads, and glutes, your upper body is involved too. The shoulders, forearms, and pecs are all taxed when you push yourself with the rope.

The use of the rope is more comprehensive in Aerobox than in a fighter's regimen. A professional boxer gets paid to jump rope. If it's boring, he puts up with it. Aerobox aims at giving you a good time while getting you fit.

It's why Aerobox provides so many rope-skipping variations and why there's more emphasis here than in a fighter's program on cultivating both feet, making you adept at skipping as nimbly off your left foot as your right. That ambidexterity—alien to a fighter's objectives—is necessary in Aerobox, for it allows you to do the more complex rope variations easily.

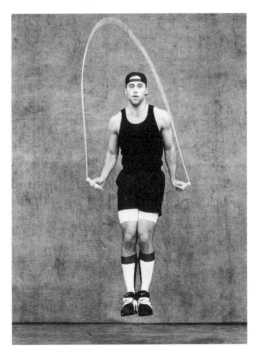

OLAJIDÉ ON THE JUMP ROPE

Traditionally, pro fighters skip rope at the end of their workouts—after the shadow boxing, bag punching, sit-ups, and sparring.

I never could figure why the rope work went last. What was the thinking that had led boxing men to view it as the finishing touch on a hard day's work?

For me, it always seemed more logical to use the rope at the beginning of a workout. Serious rope work makes demands on the cardiovascular system. I felt that if I were to do my bag punching and sparring after skipping rope, I would have to work harder at it, which would enhance stamina and endurance.

Anyway. That was how it was with me through my years as a fighter. Bucking tradition, I did the rope first and let it take its toll. I figured that by introducing fatigue into the daily regimen, and overcoming it regularly, come fight night I would refuse to be tired.

In retrospect, I guess I regarded the rope as a potent conditioning tool. Not all fighters do. Some see it as an entertainment piece. Knowing how goggle-eyed civilians get at fancy rope work, they top off the day's work by giving the fans a show.

Sugar Ray Robinson, for instance, was amazing with the rope. He'd incorporate tap dancing into his skip roping. Roberto Duran would do amazing things. I've seen him do full leg squats while turning the rope.

But like I say, their idea was to use the rope as a diversion at the end of a grueling gym session. It worked for them. Robinson and Duran are boxing legends. And my approach worked for me. I hadn't their natural gifts as fighters, but I was never beaten by fatigue.

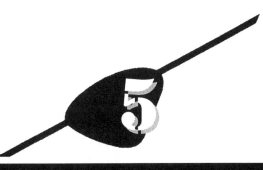

BODY TONING / ABDOMINALS

(muscles worked: for sit-ups—abdominals, obliques/ for push-ups—pectorals, deltoids, latissimus dorsi, biceps, triceps, and rotator cuffs)

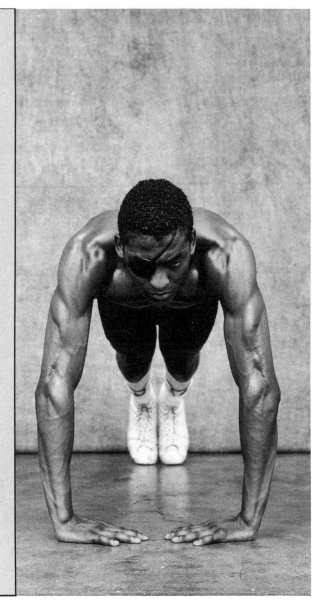

There are no high-priced weight machines in Aerobox. In this format you are working with your body's own weight.

What that means is that the common push-up becomes your basic body-toning exercise, done with uncommon variety to keep your interest level high.

Push-ups fit with Aerobox's objectives—to make you fit and give you sinewy muscles. If you are seeking to bulk up, and look like an NFL blocking guard, well, you just may want to hit the weight racks and the Cybex machines.

But in Aerobox, a variety of push-ups is what gets your body toned. The push-up works the pecs, deltoids biceps, triceps, and rotator cuffs. Fingertip push-ups—because you're elevated—accentuate the demands on the pectoral muscles and, of course,

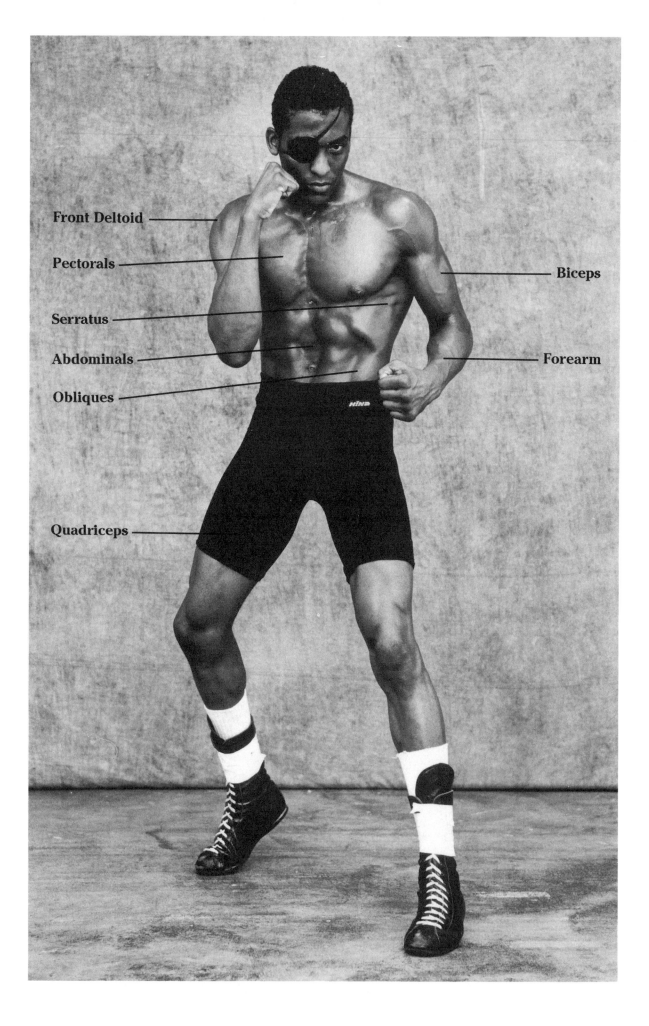

Front Deltoid

Pectorals

Serratus

Abdominals

Obliques

Quadriceps

Biceps

Forearm

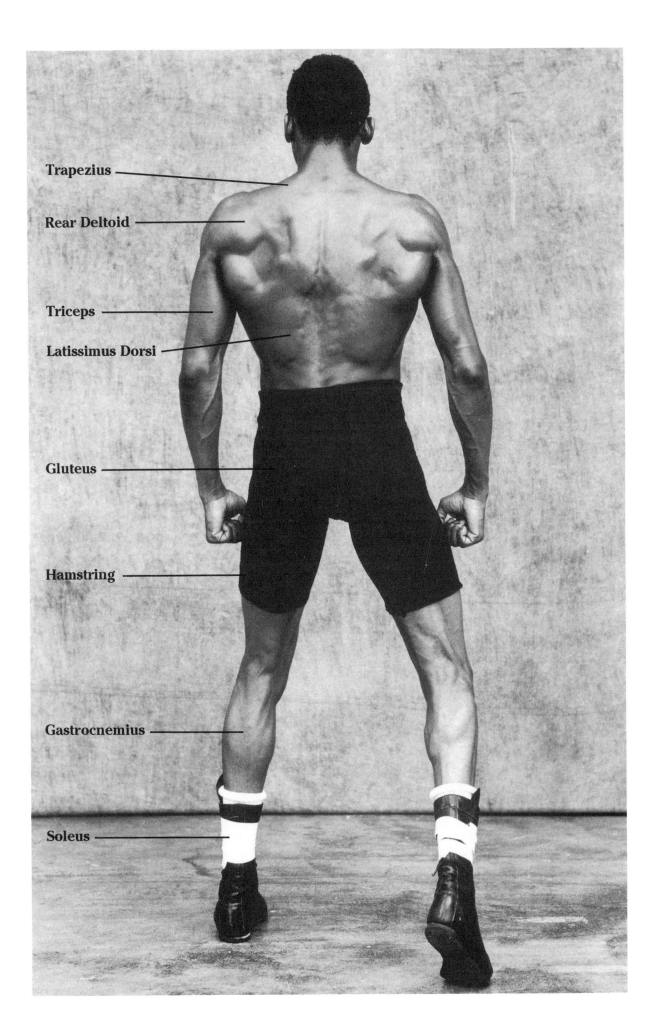

Trapezius

Rear Deltoid

Triceps

Latissimus Dorsi

Gluteus

Hamstring

Gastrocnemius

Soleus

strengthen the muscles around the metacarpals in the hands. For those who view Aerobox as a complement to recreational sparring, the fingertip push-ups will make your hands a lot stronger.

In Aerobox, you will become acquainted with the standard military push-up (palms flat, hands shoulder width apart), those fingertip push-ups, one-armed push-ups, and variations thereof.

Push-ups not only don't make you bulky, but they allow you to push yourself to the max.

Sit-ups are another way Aerobox uses your body as an exercise instrument.

It's not late-breaking news that sit-ups build your abs and that the abs are essential to a body's ability to perform. If you have a firm, strong abdomen, it enhances your ability to run, lift, bend, and twist. In boxing, the abs energize the torque a fighter needs for punches driven off the back foot—power blows like the hook, uppercut, and straight right hand. Good abs also help a fighter withstand the opponent's body punches.

Whether in sport or your daily routine, in practically everything you do the abs are involved. They are at the center of your body's universe.

As with the body-toning push-ups, Aerobox uses a variety of sit-ups to keep your mind—and energy—engaged.

Just as important is the stress placed—as with punches and movement—on proper form. That means making sure you don't do cheater's sit-ups—sit-ups in which you incorporate muscles other than the abs to help you. The home remedy for those who do is to insist they keep their fingertips on the floor, which tends to coax proper form.

The push-ups and sit-ups are the finishing touches in a cardiovascular workout that not only works the total body but does it with enough diversity to hold your attention span.

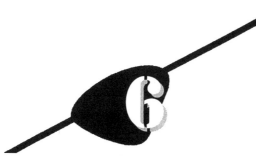

LIMBERING AND STRETCHING

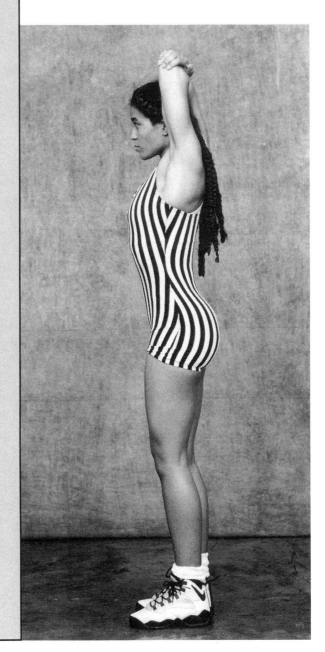

Aerobox builds bodies ... but not to the breaking point.

It's common knowledge that exercise taxes muscles and that by stretching you make sure those muscles don't break down.

The idea, of course, is to elongate muscle—both before you plunge into the workout and at the end of a session when the muscles may have grown tight.

In Aerobox, we do not do extensive stretching at the beginning of the workout. That's because the movements a fighter makes are not as alien to the body as, say, throwing a baseball or serving a tennis ball.

When you throw a punch it's within the range of everyday motions—a straight right hand is a bit like reaching for a glass of water. So instead of deep stretches we use the first few minutes of Aerobox to warm the muscles by executing our punches slowly, in a by-the-numbers manner. Then top it with some static stretches.

This adheres, philosophically, to the way fighters in a gym go about their training. Most professional boxers ease into their workout, shadow boxing at a snail's pace and then building intensity as they acquire a sweat.

At the end of an Aerobox workout—a different story. All the major muscle groups need to be stretched, in depth. This should take between six to nine minutes and relieve whatever tautness the muscles have.

Stretching is not an act to be undertaken on automatic pilot. Too many people who give maximum effort on their workout grow sloppy when it comes to stretching. Bad mistake.

For stretching done haphazardly can blow the benefits of your workout. Or, if done incorrectly—if, say, you bounce when you stretch or if you nudge cold, inflexible muscles too hard—it can do your body harm.

So don't hurry your stretches. Give them the same laser focus you would each exercise. Do your stretches slowly, and breathe naturally. Feel those muscles of yours and proceed accordingly.

When all your exercises are done, stay attentive to this final chore—the warm-down stretches. If you grow lax, you risk ending up out of commission because of an injury, and cursing yourself for neglecting a proper stretching routine.

It's no fun to be sidelined. Less so when it could have been avoided. Pay attention to your body: give it the attention it needs and it will repay you many times over.

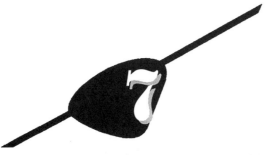

FAMOUS LAST WORDS

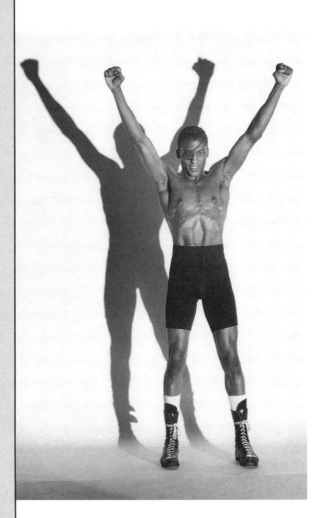

A training regimen is hard work. There's no way around that. If Aerobox has the distinction of variety—punching, footwork, skip roping, and body toning—still you cannot succeed unless you make Aerobox a habit, and this book your dog-eared companion.

When he was active, former heavyweight champion Evander Holyfield put in long days of training. He'd spar, lift weights, run, and do aerobic exercises. On one of those demanding days, he paused in the midst of a workout and, drawing deep breaths, without prompting said this of his regimen to a reporter: "It's hard but it's right."

Then he thought a moment and decided that that didn't quite get it. So he tried again.

"It's hard," he said, "but it's fair."

Hard but fair. The perfect expression of a work ethic geared for results. You wouldn't go far wrong to bring that spirit to Aerobox.

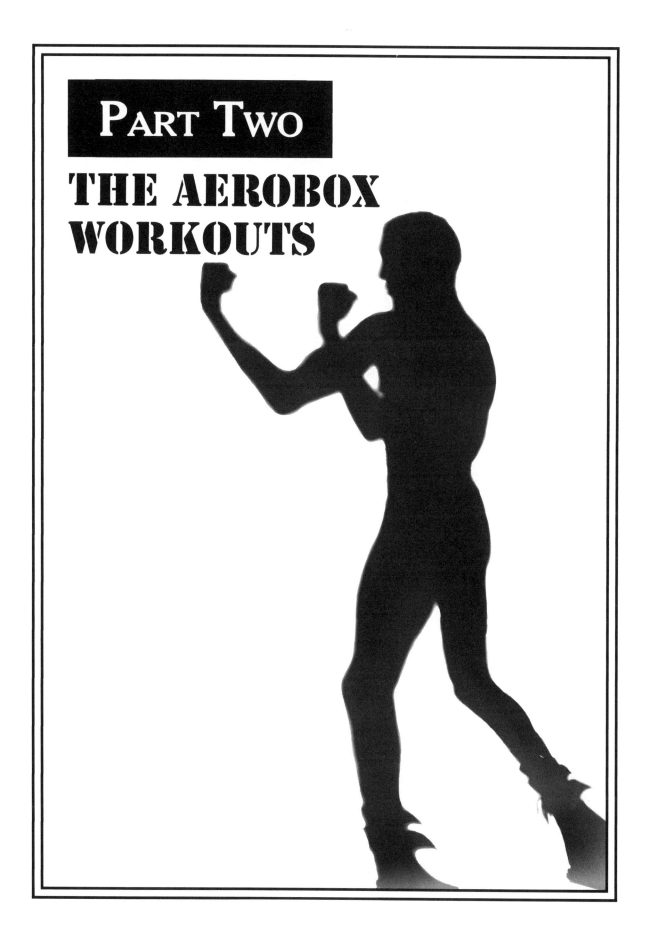

PART TWO

THE AEROBOX WORKOUTS

MIND OVER MATTER

One afternoon, when I was just starting out as an amateur boxer, I got nailed while sparring with another beginner, Nelson Ali.

Nelson was a strong kid from the Fiji Islands, with keen instincts for the sport. He hit me with a flurry of punches that left me so dazed that it took a while for me to figure out name, rank, and serial number.

It was a discouraging moment. We had both begun training in my father's gym at about the same time. To be whupped that badly that early into the game showed me I had a long way to go.

But I was determined to do better. I was fifteen at the time, and I told myself, "I'm going to get this guy back. This isn't the end of it."

Well, over the next few years, I was as dedicated to my sport as a monk is to the Scriptures. I was in the gym every day and never looked for shortcuts.

Nelson trained too, but not with

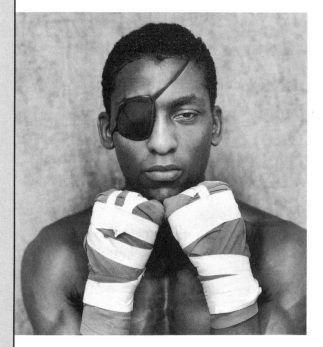

the consistency that I did. Slowly but surely the talent gap between us narrowed. And even though he was still somewhat the bigger man, that size advantage no longer gave him the edge he'd first had. In fact, on an afternoon nearly four years after he'd knocked me senseless, I returned the favor. In a sparring session, I hit him with a series of punches that had him, as they say, out on his feet.

It was a satisfying moment for me. Not so much for the payback—though that was damn nice—but rather for the affirmation it was of a work ethic my father had instilled in me.

The point of this ought to be clear enough for those of you about to undertake the rigors of Aerobox. Stick with it. Do not let those early missteps discourage you. Remember: most of the professional fighters who look so smooth in the ring have a God-given talent for boxing just as great musicians or painters do for their work. You may not possess that natural ability but with a disciplined approach you can feel the pride of accomplishment—in this case, of getting fit. So if you are awkward and undertrained when you start, don't let it defeat you. Picture what you can be. Then become it ... through consistent, focused effort.

Do not expect the miracle cure. Fitness isn't an overnight phenomenon. Be prepared to work steadily over the long haul, setting goals and then adjusting them to challenge yourself all over again.

Have faith in your commitment. Do not let what others say deter you—even well-meaning friends who just haven't the conviction you do.

I encountered negative feedback of that sort early in my career. It was November 1983. I was nineteen years old, undefeated in my first eight bouts and a professional for nearly two years. My opponent was Stacy McSwain, whose record the night we fought was seven wins, six losses, and a draw. Not a very distinguished record, but McSwain was no chump as a fighter. A year earlier, he had lost a close decision to a boxer named Sumbu Kalambay, who would go on to become a world champion.

Although I did not have an easy time of it against McSwain, I did manage to win by decision. A few days later, a businessman who worked out in my father's gym saw me and said, "How do you expect to become a world-ranked fighter if you have trouble with this kind of guy?"

He didn't say it to be nasty. It was what he honestly felt. His problem was he didn't recognize that while McSwain had a so-so record, he was an experienced fighter compared to me. For me, the match was a good test, one of many I would face on the way to a top-ten ranking and eventually two shots at a world title.

I didn't bother to explain all that to him. Opinions are like cheap suits: lots of guys have them. I was confident in my own sense of where I was and what I was destined to accomplish. And that ought to be your approach to Aerobox. Don't let the wisecracks or well-meaning cautions keep you from making progress. Trust your own sense of what is possible—and what you believe you can achieve. And go after it.

REALITY CHECK

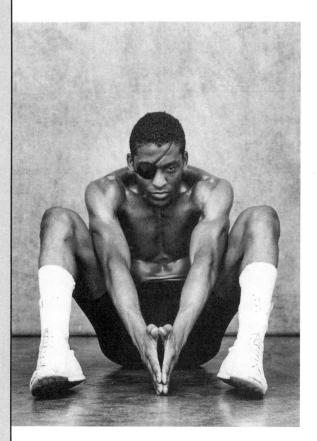

If you work hard at Aerobox, in time you will acquire the technique and finesse of a fighter while getting yourself into top physical condition.

But let's be honest. There may be a few bumps on the road to cardiovascular fitness. I point them out not to alarm or discourage you, but so that you have a realistic picture of what to expect.

Most outsiders look at boxing and see it as a primitive skill that, on the surface, does not appear as complex as, say, the pole vault or figure skating.

Maybe so. But boxing, as you may have figured from reading this far, is hardly a snap. There is artistry to it. While just about anybody can project that punch forward, it requires more than a little discipline to execute it with authority.

Think of all the boxing movies in which Hollywood stars look so pitiful making a fighter's moves. If they—with all the resources that the film industry can muster—so often end up looking like bozos (there are the exceptions, like Stallone and De Niro) it ought to give you a pretty fair idea of the work it takes to move with a fighter's authenticity.

But know this: those movements will be using muscle groups that you probably haven't worked so hard before. That means there is a good chance that on the morning after you will be sore. Don't be alarmed. This is normal. (See pages 149–150.) That soreness comes from minute tears in the ligaments and tendons and a degree of internal swelling. The swelling is the result of fluid building up internally as your body's natural way of repairing the torn connective tissues.

That's the scientific explanation. In practical terms, you feel as though you've been slugged with a mallet in those parts of your body that have been stressed. But it's no big deal. Even accomplished athletes are susceptible to muscle soreness after trying a format new to them.

As for those of you who run regularly, or have some other conditioning routine, that's no guarantee of avoiding post-workout soreness. But the fact that you're sore does *not* mean you've done your workout incorrectly. Or that you're a pathetic physical specimen. It's just the biological process that occurs when muscles grow in strength.

I repeat: muscle soreness is normal. And Aerobox gets easier on those muscles the longer you work at it.

HEAVY BREATHING

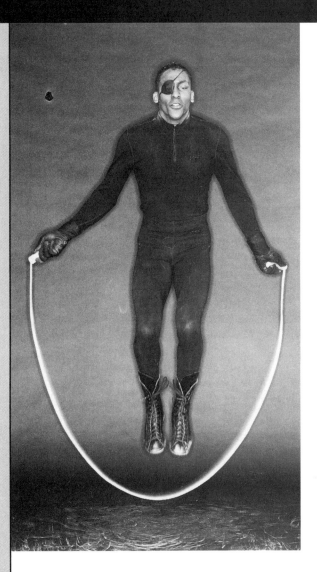

Aerobox is meant to accelerate your pulse and your breathing, and tax your body machinery.

If you are inexperienced in cardiovascular workouts, there may come a time when you feel as though your breath is being sucked out of you and your mortality is about to become an issue.

I want to prepare you for the shock of all that so you can identify the sensation and deal with it. Understand this: shortness of breath happens to experienced athletes, as it does with Aerobox beginners.

It happened to me when I fought one of my first world-class opponents, Curtis Parker, in January 1986. Typically, fighters approach the first round conservatively. That first round is what they call "a feeling-out round"—a round in which the boxers test each other's reactions with feints while gauging the distance they need to land their punches without being an easy target for a counterpunch.

Well, Parker said the hell with that and came out of his corner supercharged, throwing punches nonstop. Though I had warmed up in my dressing room, the intensity of Parker was a shock to the system. I was quickly out of my comfort zone and, for just an instant, felt a twinge of panic. "My God," I thought. "I hope the whole fight is not like this."

But—and here's the moral of the story for you—I calmed myself and dealt with it. I realized that through my intense training I was as fit as any man. So I had only to steel my mind to what was going on. Within the eye of the storm, I began to function. I met his fire with my own, figuring that once he saw he couldn't overwhelm me with his fury, he would calm down. Which he did. And before long I had my second wind and control of a fight I ended up winning by a ten-round decision.

In my Aerobox classes, I see that certain look that newcomers get when it feels like their heart is about to leap out of their chest. It's usually the rapid-fire punch-and-move sequences, or the skip rope, that brings on that discomfort and leads people to question why they are doing this to themselves. Some of them just walk out of the class, convinced this is more work than they will ever be capable of doing. They are wrong. They simply haven't learned to manage the body's more radical moments.

Aerobox was not designed to be unpleasant. Being fit is exhilarating. So listen to the voice within. If you're uncomfortable, you always have the option of slackening the pace. Work within your range. Fighters adjust in the ring. If they're fatigued, they back off from the action until they feel revived. There are tricks fighters know to make those lulls look like action. You don't need to be that creative. Just get comfortable. Aerobox is not cruel and unusual punishment. Never pursue it to the point of self-damage.

OLAJIDÉ ON THE MIND OF THE FIGHTER

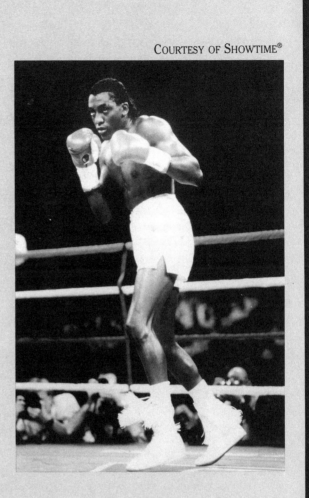

Fighters are an elite group of fit, tough men. But their success, or failure, in the ring—like yours in Aerobox—often is tied to how strong-minded and how focused they are. The mind of a fighter can empower him beyond what his body seems capable of, and it can diminish him and make his skills irrelevant.

Former heavyweight champion Evander Holyfield, for instance, had an inner toughness that made character an issue in every fight. Holyfield's training added intense weight and aerobic workouts to the more traditional boxing regimen, and was calculated to produce a boxer whose ability to fight at a furious pace was his tactical edge against often bigger and stronger men. It was the revenge of the overachiever.

On the other hand, Buster Douglas, the man Holyfield knocked out to become heavyweight champion, now stands as an object lesson in self-destruction. Douglas, you may remember, is the only man to defeat Mike Tyson, knocking him out in nine rounds in February 1990 in Tokyo. That night Douglas, a 42–1 underdog, was a fit and mentally prepared fighter. Not only did he outclass Tyson, but he just wouldn't be intimidated by Tyson, as so many opponents of Iron Mike had been in the past. In fact, at times he treated Tyson practically with contempt, hitting him after the bell and roughhousing him. He was in complete possession of the fight.

But from all reports, Douglas changed once he won the title, appointing himself the boss of his boxing regimen. That meant that Douglas's manager, John Johnson, a demanding sort who had pushed and cajoled the sometimes lethargic Douglas for the Tyson fight, was now relegated to the sidelines. A token figure. Manager in title only. Which, newsmen said, caused Douglas to revert to character. He ate too much and trained too little. From the sleek 228-pound conqueror of Tyson he swelled to 246 pounds. And offered pathetically little resistance when he fought, and lost, to Holyfield.

Often the mind games of boxing can be quite strange. In April 1986, I fought and beat a fighter named James (Hard Rock) Green. Green was a squat man, built like a tank. He had fast hands and hit hard. He had no fear. At one time he was a world-class fighter. But Green had a disturbing flaw. When an opponent managed to cut him, he came unglued. At the sight of his own blood, he floundered. He was a different man. He did not fight with the same focus. A hard-to-explain mental phenomenon.

Speaking of mental phenomena ... Roberto Duran was a world champion in several weight classes and a fighter I always admired. Most casual boxing fans remember him for his intensity—those glowing eyes and that destroyer's purposefulness. But what the average guy missed was how technically skilled, how knowledgeable Duran was in the ring. He had subtle moves that only the aficionado, or fellow professional, could appreciate.

But Duran, of course, is widely remembered for a boxing moment that got away from him, when his fighter's mind misfired, causing a baffling psychological breakdown during a bout. In November 1980, in the midst of a world title fight against Sugar Ray Leonard, Duran walked away from his opponent and told the referee, "No más," Spanish for "No more." Duran quit against a fighter he had beaten earlier in the year.

Duran later would claim that he had a stomach problem, but the press didn't buy the excuse, insisting that Duran had cracked—that his very macho character couldn't cope with the way Leonard mocked him while the fight was going on and tried to make him look silly.

The funny thing is that while the "no más" bout brought headlines and extensive coverage—and brought shame to Duran—when the two fighters fought a last time, in December 1989, there are those who insist it offered a muted version of "no más."

That night, Leonard took advantage of the fact that time had eroded Duran's quickness more than his own. Nine years after "no más," Leonard would circle Duran from a safe distance, hit him a quick shot and step away before a serious fight could get started. A conservative battle plan it was, and, some experts said, Duran's only way to offset it would have required him to lunge and chase and be a bit reckless. But these same observers depicted Duran as Robby the Robot in the mechanical quarter turns he made, this way and that, waiting and hoping Leonard would change tactics and mix it up with him.

Whether, as some critics would claim, the same macho pride that had caused Duran to bolt in 1980 was keeping him grounded nine years later ... whether Duran had chosen to save face rather than gamble for victory is hard to say. Maybe Duran was fighting with injuries. Maybe he was setting a trap that simply did not work. But all the speculation reinforces my point—that the body of a fighter does not operate on automatic pilot ... it must have a mind geared for battle.

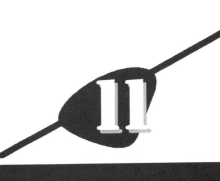
GETTING READY

WHAT TO WEAR

Now that you've gotten a kind of emotional road map to Aerobox, let's get down to practical matters.

Like what to wear. Loose-fitting clothes—a T-shirt and shorts—are what most folks go for. But if you're comfortable in aerobic outfits made from spandex or Lycra, no problem. They absorb sweat and will do just fine.

Some folks like to wear rubber suits or sweat suits to coax a bigger sweat. That would be a mistake with Aerobox, which gives you all the exercise you're going to want. Rubber suits do not allow the pores to breathe naturally. So forget gimmicky clothing. What your objective should be is to trigger changes in your metabolism through consistent exercise. That is the sensible, and lasting, way to change your body ... and to get fit.

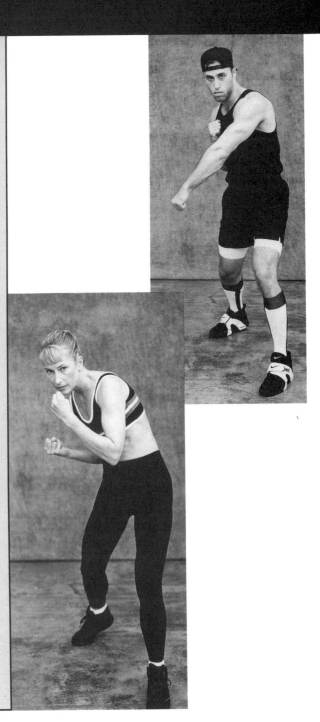

Heavy clothes that allow your pores to breath naturally are okay, particularly in a cold workout environment. If, say, a wintry blast has hit your city and left your apartment or gym too cold for comfort, then you might want to "layer up" until your body has gotten a sweat and is operating with indifference to that cold. At that point, the sweatshirt and/or windbreaker can be stripped, and so can the sweatpants if you want.

Footwear? I recommend aerobic or cross-training shoes. Hightop models give a little more ankle support, and that's a definite plus.

But hightop, or low-cut, basketball shoes are not as suited for Aerobox. Basketball shoes are heavier and, because of that, are a burden when you're using the jump rope.

Running shoes have less padding at the front of the foot than aerobic or cross-training shoes. Since so much of boxing is executed off that front portion of the foot, it diminishes the practical value of the running shoe. And with the tread that running shoes have, you risk an injury occurring if your shoe gets snagged while you are making a move.

EATING

What about eating before your workout? I like to be a little hungry when I exercise. But what suits you may be different. The thing here is to be sensible. Avoid fried foods or meals that lie heavy on your stomach. But during a workout you may, if you like, drink water whenever you feel the need to.

SETTING

Most of you will be doing your Aerobox workout at home. The preferred surface would be a flat wooden floor and a ceiling at least nine feet high. Other options: an empty indoor basketball court or an unused tennis court.

If you're thinking that the jump-roping phase of Aerobox may create a problem, think again. All you need is three feet in front of you, three feet to the rear, and that nine-foot ceiling.

Finally, music. What sound you want—and whether in fact you prefer to work out in silence—is up to you. If you choose to do your Aerobox program with musical accompaniment, your best bet is a sound with a simple steady beat so that you can punch or execute your moves on the beat. That beat can also help you regulate your skip-rope rhythm.

In my classes, I use the house music played in clubs around New York by a premiere deejay friend of mine, Lord G. These are special deejay mixes of songs not readily found on your radio dial. What the songs tend to have in common is a potent bass drum that gives you a lot of backbeat and an aggressive, driving mood.

My students constantly ask where they can get these cuts and are disheartened to learn these mixes are not available to the public. However, there are CDs that have the essence of the type of music I use. I recommend the *Orbital 2* album.

Another type of music I use is more melodic and less driven—good for our jump-rope work—and is typified by certain songs performed by Us3, like "Tukka Yoots Riddim" or "Flip Fantasia," or "Love and Happiness" by India.

While silence may be golden for some, most folks are energized by a good rhythmic sound. Music motivates. It pleases the ear, and enlivens the spirit. In the end, though, it's your choice. Whatever works for you.

The Aerobox workout is designed to be done three times a week. For ambitious sorts who exercise five, six, seven days a week, and want more Aerobox, I'd caution not to overdo it.

Aerobox provides a workout that, done with gusto, will tax your body to the max. Muscles need time to recover ... or they break down. So don't go crazy.

But if you have an athlete's capacity for work, and you're craving Aerobox, I offer this suggestion. Supplement other exercise formats with fragments of Aerobox on the other four days. For instance, after you take that step-aerobics class, do a series of skip-rope maneuvers from Aerobox. Or if your preference is the stationary bicycle, why not finish the workout with a series of push-ups from Aerobox. Or if you lift weights, try some shadow boxing after.

Whatever the level of your athleticism, you won't lack for a challenge with Aerobox. To find out just what the program can do for you, let's move on to the workouts. First, the beginner's.

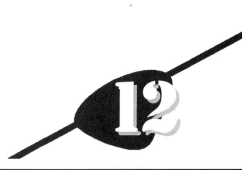

THE BEGINNER'S WORKOUT

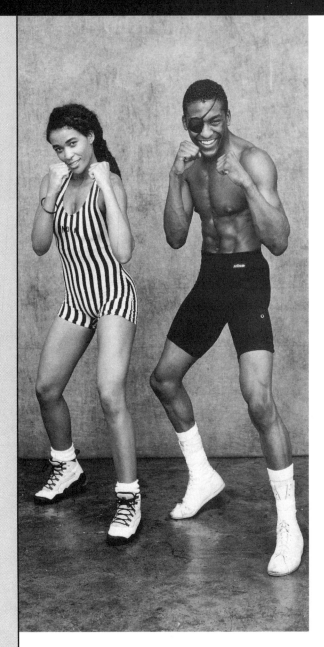

Not all athletes are created equal.

So why would it be any different for those of you seeking fun and fitness from Aerobox?

I assume the readers of this book will range from thick-waisted couch potatoes to ex-varsity athletes who have never let themselves get out of shape.

That means that for some folks Aerobox is a chance for a life change while for others it is a way to expand their fitness horizons.

Whatever the reason you've taken up Aerobox, a few guidelines for the beginner's workout apply to all of you.

Master the one-hour beginner's workout before even thinking about advanced Aerobox. Do not be deceived by the word "beginner's." When I told you earlier in these pages that former world-champion fighters have wilted trying to do Aerobox, I was not exaggerating.

That said, I urge you to try every Aerobox exercise. You may not get it just right the first time, but you lay the groundwork for future progress. Try, try, try. Shoot for small gains, maintaining written records if that helps motivate you.

But keep it all in perspective. The rhythms of boxing, the diversity of movements and skills make Aerobox satisfying, even fun . . . so long as you work to your skill level. Work hard, but don't push beyond what you're capable of. Let's begin . . .

WARM-UPS

OBJECTIVE: To raise your heart rate to a level at which you can do Aerobox effectively. To alert the upper and lower body to the sort of movements that will be incorporated in the exercises you will subsequently do over the next hour. To alert the muscles to exercise and make them somewhat more injury-proof.

SHOULDER SHRUGS
(with and without toe raises)

POSITION: Assume a boxer's stance—left foot forward, right foot back . . . (see pages 7–8).

MOVEMENT: Drop your hands to your sides. Push up from the balls of your feet for 16 toe raises. Now rotate the shoulders in a circular and forward motion 16 times. Then reverse direction for another 16 shoulder shrugs while simultaneously rising up on your toes with each shoulder shrug to work the calves.

MUSCLES WORKED: Calves, soleus, trapezius, and the muscles of the feet and ankle.

TORSO TWISTS
(with and without punching)

POSITION: The boxer's stance.

MOVEMENT: Right-handed stance: rotate your body to the right on the count of one; come back to center and rotate your body to the left on the count of two. Repeat without stopping for a count of 32.

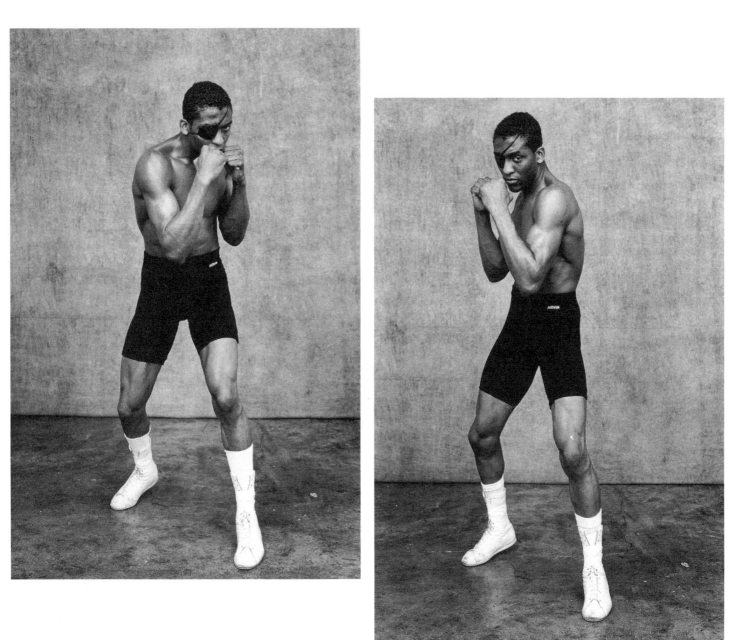

THE REST OF THE SEQUENCE: Begin another 32 torso twists. But as you twist right on the count of one, punch with your left hand—a flicking motion directed across your body and downward, with the wrist getting turned and the punch synchronized to your body's rotation.

Now switch to a left-handed stance and rotate left and right for 32 counts . . . and then do a second 32-count set in which you punch as you twist.

REMEMBER: Rather than releasing the punch from set position, in this exercise hold your hands at the chest or upper abdomen. On retracting the punch, the hands go back to mid-torso rather than to set position. When you rotate to either side, and you throw your punch, it's a casual thrust, as though you're tossing a small ball against the ground. Keep your shoulders rounded, chin down, and knees bent. Feet firmly grip the ground. This protects the lower back from strain. Don't let your knees sway.

MUSCLES WORKED: Waist and oblique muscles and those of the shoulder region.

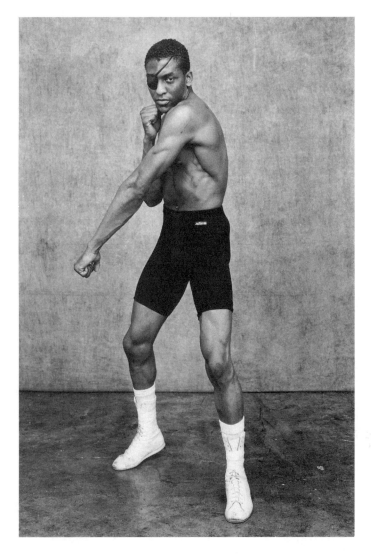

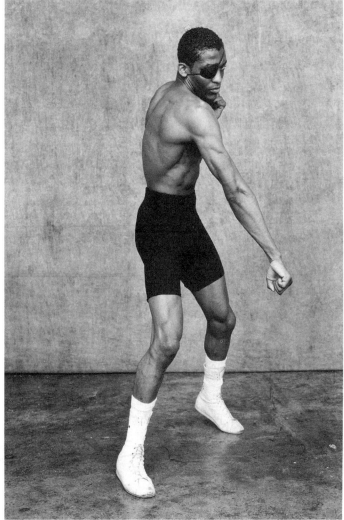

Left-hand stance—southpaw

SLIP TWIST-AND-PUNCH

POSITION: The southpaw boxer's stance (see page 8).

MOVEMENT: On the count of one, tilt sideways from the waist to the right and then back to center. On the count of two, to the left and back to center. This is a 32-count set, executed at a speed one level above slow motion. It's a tic-toc motion that alerts the obliques and gets them oriented. Repeat from a right-handed stance for 32 counts.

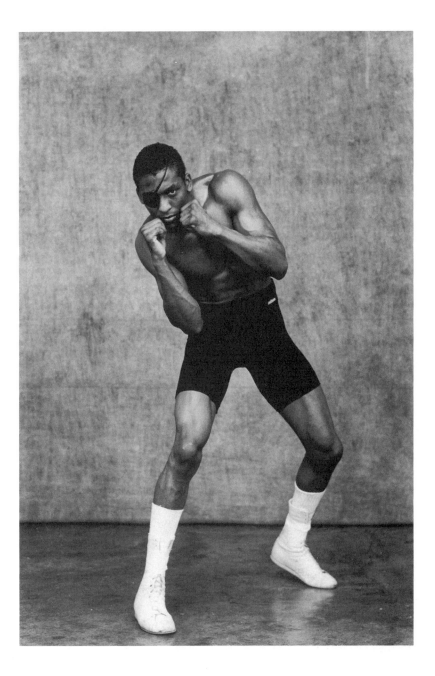

THE REST OF THE SEQUENCE: Still in your right-handed stance, slip punches by bending from the knees, being sure to keep your chin tucked in. Roll under to the left. Straighten. That's the count of one. Roll under to the right. Straighten. That's the count of two. Repeat for 32 counts. Then, from a southpaw stance, do another 32-count set.

Still in that southpaw stance, do 16 torso twists, rotating to the left first and then to the right.

That's followed by torso twists accompanied by that flicking punch down on each rotation—the right hand as you twist left, the left hand as you twist right. Again for 16 counts.

Repeat the twist-and-synchronized-punch for 16 counts, but elevate the arc of your punches. Rather than flicking them down, your trajectory is across your shoulders, as though you're seeking a good shoulder stretch. Do not stand straight up. Keep the shoulders rounded. Be sure to twist as you throw your punches: it intensifies the work the abs have to do and lessens the strain on the lower back.

Still as a southpaw—and without accentuating the torso twist—throw straight punches, sixteen in all, alternating right and left hands.

Now assume a right-handed stance, and repeat the 16-count sets you just did as a lefty: sideways twists, twist and punch downward, twist and punch shoulder level, and finally straight punches.

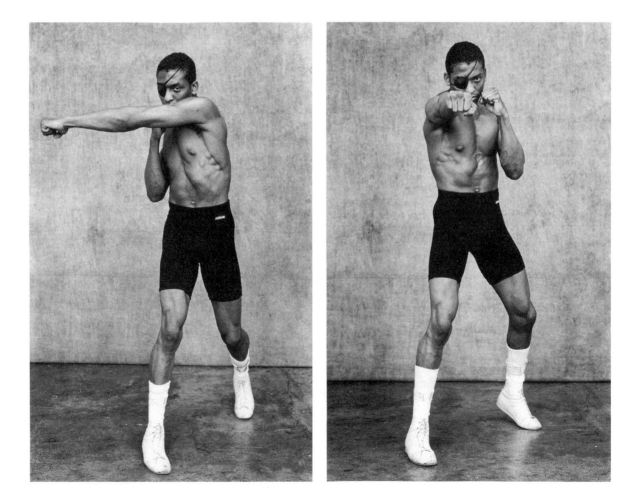

REMEMBER: When you slip punches by bending at the knees, your objective is to create a sweeping U or V motion. Do not bend with your back. Strictly the knees. The emphasis here is on the glutes and thighs, and you're working at a moderate pace. At those points in the V-slip where you straighten, never lock your knees.

One other point. As you slip from side to side, don't let your hands get caught up in the rhythm and swing wide of your body. Keep those fists in set position.

MUSCLES WORKED: Quads, glutes, obliques, and shoulder region.

At this point in the beginner's workout, you will do a series of light stretches for both the upper and lower body.

SHOULDER STRETCH

POSITION: While standing with your feet shoulder-width apart, place your left arm across your chest. Put your right arm beneath the left and perpendicular to it so that you are cradling the left arm at the lower end of the right bicep.

MOVEMENT: Using the right arm, pull the left toward you and hold it there for a count of 8. You should feel the stretch at the back of the shoulders. Now reverse the position of your arms, and stretch the shoulder muscles on the other side of your body, again for that count of 8.

MUSCLES WORKED: The back, shoulder blades, rear deltoids, upper triceps.

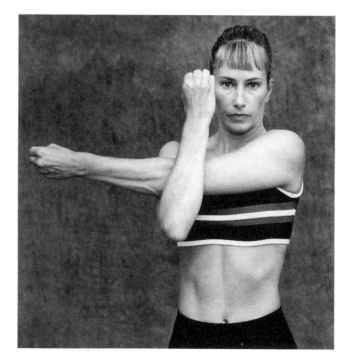

TRICEPS STRETCH

POSITION: Stand with your feet shoulder-width apart. Point your right elbow to the ceiling and place the fingertips of your right hand between the shoulder blades. With your left hand, you grip the right elbow.

MOVEMENT: Push the upright portion of the right arm backward and hold for a count of 8. Your right hand should slide down your back. Now reverse the position of the arms, and stretch the left triceps, again for that count of 8.

MUSCLES WORKED: Triceps, lats.

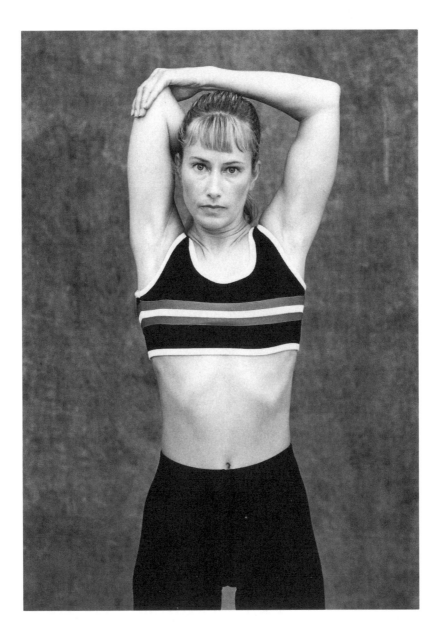

CALF STRETCH

POSITION: You're in a modified boxer's stance, your right foot back, your left foot forward, with the left knee bent and the toes pointing straight ahead. The right leg should be straight. The space between the legs is somewhat exaggerated. For me, a six-footer, the distance is two feet.

MOVEMENT: From that position, you lean with both hands on top of the left thigh, the right hand covering the left hand. Now push that right heel to the ground for a count of 10 to stretch the calves. Then reverse sides for the same count.

MUSCLES WORKED: Gastrocnemius, soleus.

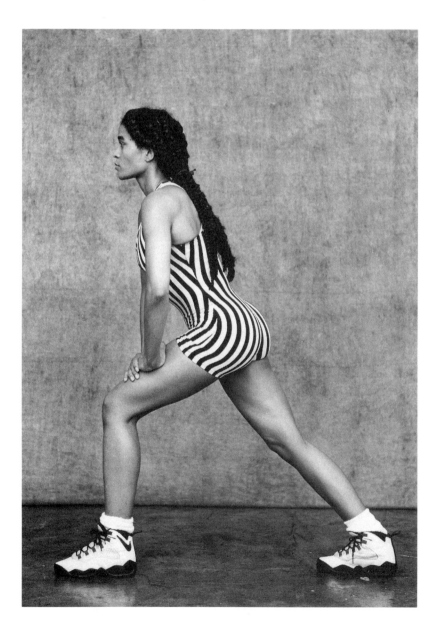

HAMSTRING STRETCH

POSITION: Assume the boxer's stance—left foot forward, right to the rear.

MOVEMENT: Lift the toes of your left foot, pointing them upward and keeping the heel of that foot in contact with the floor. Stick your rear end out and lower yourself by bending from the waist while both your hands rest on your left knee. Your chin must be up. As you lower, you will look like a baseball pitcher leaning forward and peering in to the catcher for signals. Hold for a count of 10 and feel the stretch in your hamstrings. Repeat from the opposite side.

MUSCLES WORKED: Hamstrings.

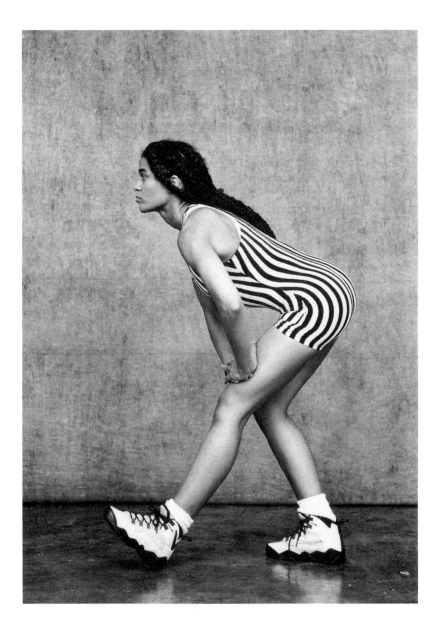

ANKLE LOOSENER

POSITION: The boxer's stance.

MOVEMENT: Point the toe of your rear foot (the right foot) to the ground. Roll that foot over the big toe and second toe in a clockwise motion for a count of 8. Then a counterclockwise motion for a count of 8. Switch sides and roll the left foot in the same manner and count.

THE REST OF THE SEQUENCE: At the completion of this stretch, reverse your stance: put your right foot forward and left to the rear, and repeat the sequence of calf, hamstring, and ankle stretches from the position.

MUSCLES WORKED: Jumping rope and nonstationary boxing moves require a lot of movement from the ankles. This stretch prepares the ankle joint for them.

   With these simple limbering maneuvers, you are now ready to start the punching phase of beginner's Aerobox.

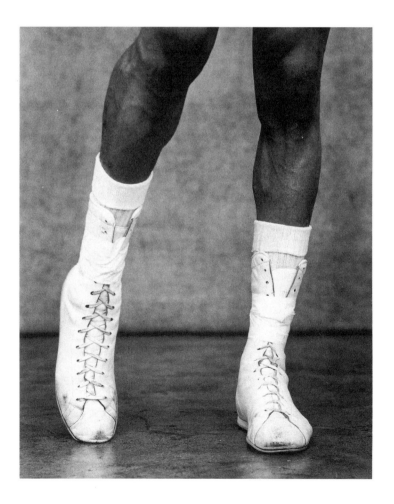

PUNCHING

OBJECTIVE: To master the techniques of boxing's basic punches and execute them, ultimately, in rapid-fire sequences.

THE JAB

KEY ELEMENTS:

1. Prior to releasing the jab, don't lift the elbow. By doing so, you alert the opponent to the jab that is about to come. This is called telegraphing a punch.
2. The punch comes from the shoulder; do not snap the elbow.
3. Retract to set position once the punch is thrown.

POSITION: Assume a fighter's stance, your left foot leading.

MOVEMENT: Begin by throwing the jab in slow motion. This serves to alert the muscles and to track the proper trajectory of the punch. It's a four-count movement. The jab goes out on one, back to set position on two, and you count three-four. Do this four-count set 4 times.

THE REST OF THE SEQUENCE: Now we accelerate the velocity. The punch goes out and is retracted on one, then you count two-three-four. Do this four-count set 4 times.

In the next stage, the movements are even more forceful. The jab is thrown and retracted on one, and again on two, then count three-four. This four-count set is done 4 times.

Now jab and retract on one, again on two, and still again on three. Then count four. Repeat this set 4 times.

In your final set, you jab and retract 8 times without pausing. That's one set. Do 4 sets in all.

Note: For your second workout, you will do all these exercises for the jab as a left-hander.

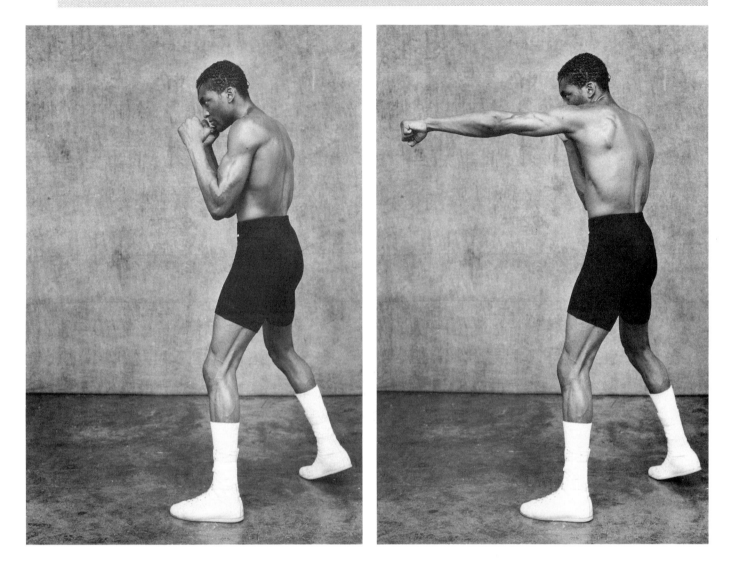

REMEMBER: As you're working the jab, visualize an opponent and imagine your contact point. Concentrate on proper form, but don't let the jab "hang" out there. Bring it back as quickly as you shoot it out. Fighters who throw a "lazy" jab—the vernacular for a jab not taken back to set position immediately—are asking for trouble. Smart opponents take note of the lazy jab and time their right hand to land on the jaw, at just the point where the retracted glove should be.

As with all punches, the exercise benefits come from extending the arm. Get the hands away from the face, and let your punches go. No half punches.

Don't extend your arm past 95 percent on the jab. Visualize making contact with the knuckles of the index and middle fingers. Keep the nonpunching arm close to your body, its fist protecting your jaw.

MUSCLES WORKED: Delts, pecs, triceps, biceps, traps.

THE RIGHT-HAND POWER PUNCH

KEY ELEMENTS:

1. As you throw the right, rotate your shoulders and keep your abs tight.
2. Your legs are semitense; your feet grip the ground as you transfer weight forward.
3. When the punch is delivered, the bottom of your fist is parallel to the ground and you retract the punch with the same intensity you delivered it.

POSITION: Assume a fighter's stance.

MOVEMENT: Begin by throwing the right hand in slow motion. The punch goes out on one, back on two, count three-four. Do 4 sets.

THE REST OF THE SEQUENCE: Accelerate the punch. Your right hand shoots forward on one, is retracted on two, count three-four. Four sets.

With even more forceful movements the right is delivered and withdrawn on one, and again on two, count three-four. This sequence is done 4 times.

Finally, punch and retract on one, and again on two and three, then count four. Do 8 sets.

REMEMBER: It is important to get that torque into the punch. No torque, no power.

MUSCLES WORKED: Abs, traps, lats, pecs, triceps, and upper back.

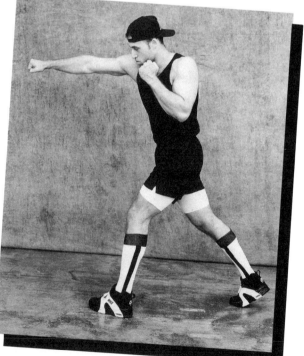

THE LEFT HOOK

KEY ELEMENTS:

1. With your elbow shoulder high, the left goes out and across the body.
2. Don't swing the elbow back for a head start; drive the punch from the shoulder.
3. As you start the punch, swing your left shoulder back slightly, then rotate it forward as you let the hook go.

POSITION: Assume a fighter's stance.

MOVEMENT: Begin by throwing the left hook in slow motion. The left goes out on one, back on two, and you count three-four. Do 4 sets.

THE REST OF THE SEQUENCE: Accelerate the punch. The hook goes out and back on one, count two-three-four. Four sets.

With more forceful movements throw your hook and retract it on one, and again on two, then count three-four. Repeat this through 4 sets.

Finally, hook and retract on one, and again on two and three, then count four. Eight sets.

REMEMBER: Your imagined impact point is slightly past your nose. Do not let the punch go beyond there. The bottom of the fist faces you when the punch is delivered.

MUSCLES WORKED: Biceps, obliques, and upper back.

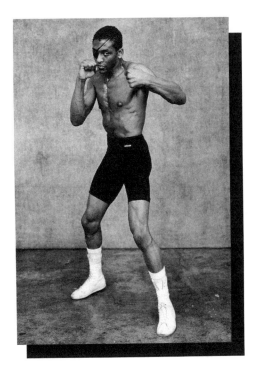

THE RIGHT UPPERCUT

KEY ELEMENTS:

1. Rotate the fist up and stop the punch at face level, with the palm of your hand facing you.
2. Twist the upper body when throwing the punch.
3. Retract your fist to set position.

POSITION: Assume a fighter's stance.

MOVEMENT: Begin by throwing the right uppercut in slow motion. The punch is driven upward on one, retracted on two, you count three-four. Do 4 sets.

THE REST OF THE SEQUENCE: Accelerate the uppercut. Shoot it out and bring it back on one, and again on two, count three-four. Four sets.

   With more forceful movements the uppercut is delivered and retracted on one, and again on two and three, then count four. Repeat this sequence 4 times.

   Finally, throw the uppercut and retract on all four beats, then count one, two, three-four. That constitutes a set. Do 8 sets.

REMEMBER: Keep the legs semitense and twist up with your upper body. Do not bounce up and down with your knees to help the punch out. Discipline yourself.

MUSCLES WORKED: Lats, obliques, traps, and biceps.

   We are now ready to try more advanced punching sequences, some of which involve the slipping techniques we learned earlier (see pages 23–26).

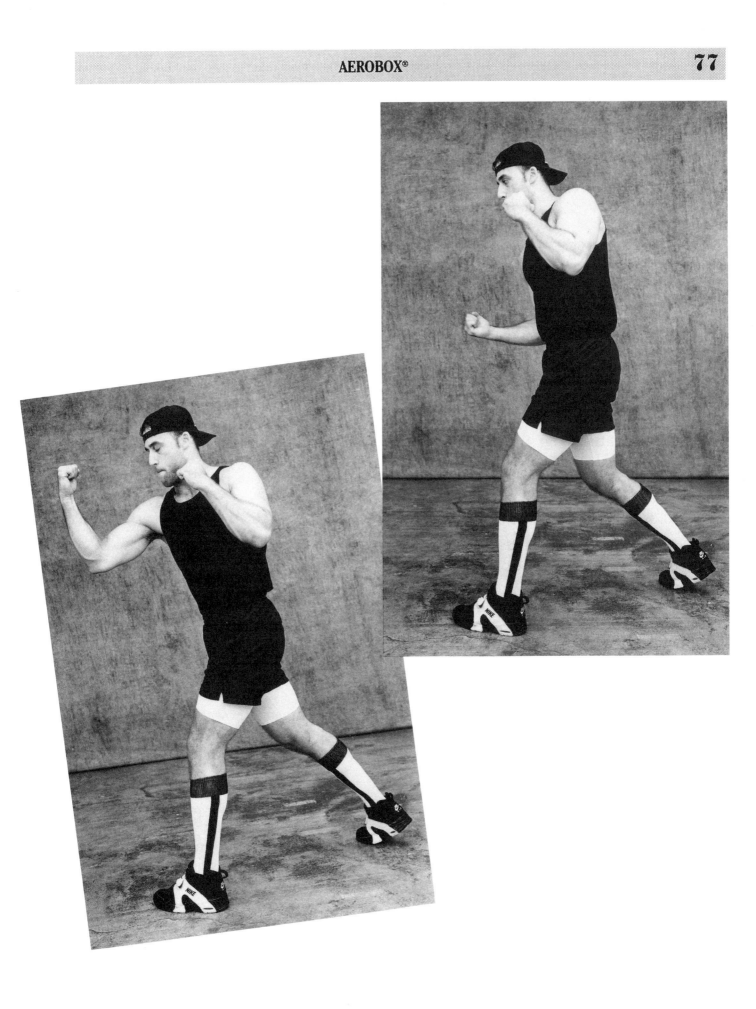

SLIPS AND COUNTERS

OBJECTIVE: To combine punching techniques with the defensive maneuvers a fighter employs.

LATERAL SLIPS AND COUNTERS

POSITION: Assume a fighter's stance.

MOVEMENT: Slip sideways to your left, bending from the waist, then return to center before firing a quick left jab. That's the count of one. Then slip right, come back to center and throw a right hand. That's the count of two. Repeat for 16 counts. The velocity of your punches should be a level up from slow motion.

REMEMBER: Be sure to complete your defensive movement before you throw your punch. There is a tendency among beginners to abbreviate the slip in their haste to uncork the punches.

MUSCLES WORKED: Obliques, pecs, deltoids, traps, and muscles of the upper back.

V-SLIPS AND COUNTERS

POSITION: Assume a fighter's stance.

MOVEMENT: Bending from your knees, slip to your left and throw the left hook (count of one), then slip to your right and throw a straight right (count of two). Repeat until you reach 16 counts. The velocity of the punches is a level up from slow motion.

THE REST OF THE SEQUENCE: Repeat the previously executed lateral slips and counters and V-slips and counters. For 8 sets each, and for 4 sets each. Then . . .
   Slip left from the waist and jab, slip right from the waist and throw a straight right hand. Do a V-slip to the left and hook, then a V-slip to the right and throw a power right. That's followed by a 16-punch power barrage of left-right, left-right. All that constitutes one set. Do 4 sets.

MUSCLES WORKED: Obliques, lats, delts, pecs, triceps, biceps, upper back, traps, glutes, and quads.

COMBINATION PUNCHING

OBJECTIVE: To utilize the basic punches in complex series. To raise your heart rate and enhance your coordination. To build upper body strength and sharpen muscle definition.

POSITION: Assume a fighter's stance.

MOVEMENT: Jab at a velocity a level above slow motion. Then execute a double left jab with more intensity. Follow with a double jab and a right, then a double jab, a right and left hook. That makes up one set. Do 4 sets.

THE REST OF THE SEQUENCE: The next combination punching sequence is even more intense. Begin with a double jab, a right and a left, executed rapidly. Repeat 8 times.

Your final series is even more intricate. Begin with 1) a jab, then 2) jab and slip to the left from the waist, then 3) jab and slip to the left from the waist and throw the left hook. On 4), you repeat jab-slip-left-hook and add a right uppercut. On 5), you repeat jab-slip-left-hook-right-uppercut and add another left hook. On 6), you add a straight right hand to the previous sequence.

Do steps one through six 4 times, then do step six rapidly 8 times.

MUSCLES WORKED: All muscles of the upper body and glutes, quads, and midsection.

By this point, your heart should be pumping and you ought to be lathered up with a good sweat. But don't pat yourself on the back just yet. For that skip rope that you are about to take in hand can be as tough on a body as a medieval torture rack. That's a joke. Sort of.

THE ROPE

OBJECTIVE: To master the techniques of jumping rope and then to employ the rope to take you to your aerobic threshold. The benefits? Total body coordination, increased agility, stamina, body tone and definition, and fat loss.

Prior to the workout, make sure you measure your skip rope so that there's no time wasted once you get into beginner's Aerobox (see pages 30–31).

Remember: no child-type plastic ropes. You want a serious workout rope. The inferior ropes turn too slowly and force you to jump higher. That leaves you susceptible to injury.

So does jumping barefoot. Leave your training shoes on.

If you've never jumped rope before, this phase of Aerobox may not be easy. Not only will you have plenty to think about regarding technique, but the demands on your cardiovascular system from the rope compound the difficulty.

Do the best you can. Those students of mine who stick with it invariably get the hang of the rope. It's simply a matter of putting the time in. Like the out-of-towner who accosted a hard-boiled New Yorker and asked, "How do I get to Carnegie Hall?" The same answer applies here. Practice, practice, practice.

SIDE-TO-SIDE FIGURE EIGHTS
(with and without basic jumps)

KEY ELEMENTS:

1. Grip the rope by the handles. Do not grab the rope itself. If the rope is too long, tie a slip knot.
2. Left hand on top, roll your wrists to the right, then to the left. Keep the hands close together but never let them cross over each other.
3. Your objective: let the rope make an X in front of you, and loops at the side.

POSITION: Assume a squared-off stance, your feet three to four inches apart.

MOVEMENT: Begin by swinging the rope slowly side to side, creating your figure eights (see page 31). You swing the rope to the left first one day and to the right first the next day. Do those side-to-side configurations 16 times to create the momentum for your basic jump.

THE REST OF THE SEQUENCE: Without any pause, go from your figure eights into the basic jump for 16 revolutions. Then do 8 slow figure eights, followed by the basic jump for 16 more revolutions, turning the rope one revolution per jump. All that constitutes a set. Do 2 sets.

REMEMBER: On the basic jump, your hands are in front of your body, elbows close to the waist. Turn the rope from waist level, with your wrists rotating forward. Don't kick your heels backward when you jump; adapt the soft-shoe approach. Push from the toes. Concentrate on form. Don't hurry. If you feel awkward, just jump without counting.

MUSCLES WORKED: Forearms, traps, thighs, calves, soleus, delts, pecs, the muscles of your feet, and your cardiovascular system.

REPRISE: Swing the rope side to side 8 times, then do 32 basic jumps. Then swing the rope side to side 16 times at double the pace, and do 16 basic jumps. Now you're ready for ...

ONE-FOOTED HOPS

POSITION: Square off your stance and grip the rope by the handles.

MOVEMENT: On this exercise, one foot is always off the ground while the other foot hops. Start with 4 jumps, one per revolution, on the right foot, then 4 on the left. Do 32 revolutions of the rope—16 jumps on each foot.

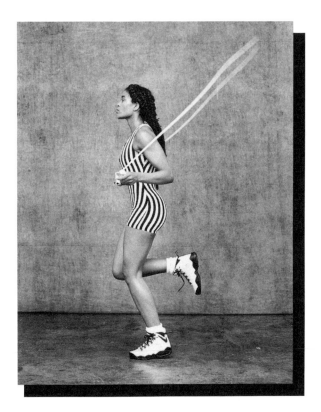

REMEMBER: The push comes from the ball of the foot, with the knees slightly bent. Do not bend the knees too much or "buck forward" with the body. Keep your weight centered. Don't throw your chin up. Not too straight a back either. Jumps like this one lay the groundwork for more complex maneuvers to follow and teach you to control separate muscles selectively.

MUSCLES WORKED: Same as in the basic jump, with calves and soleus muscles accentuated.

REPRISE: Do 8 basic jumps. Then swing the rope slowly side to side 16 times, taking measured breaths as you do. Finish with 8 more basic jumps. That sets you up for . . .

DOWNHILL JUMPS

POSITION: Square off your stance and grip the rope by the handles.

MOVEMENT: The upper body stays in place while, with feet together, the lower body swings side to side on each jump. The motion is like the pendulum of a grandfather clock, or the slalom moves of a champion skier. Do 32 revolutions in all, one jump per revolution.

REMEMBER: Be aware of your hands as you turn the rope. They should be at waist level, just above the belt line. Don't jump too wide. Stay low to the ground, especially if you are not wearing cross-training or aerobic shoes.

MUSCLES WORKED: The same muscles as in the basic jump, with the glutes, quads, lateral buttocks, hips, and calves accentuated.

REPRISE: Do 8 basic jumps. Then swing the rope slowly side to side 16 times, taking those measured breaths. Finish with 8 more basic jumps as your lead-in to . . .

PIVOT JUMPS

POSITION: Square off your stance and grip the rope by the handles.

MOVEMENT: On the count of one, turn sideways to the left as you jump. On two, come back to the center. On three, turn sideways to the right. On four, back to the center. Repeat the four-count maneuver 8 times. That constitutes one set. Do 8 sets.

REMEMBER: The feet stay together and the heel of the foot still doesn't touch the ground.

MUSCLES WORKED: The same muscles as in the basic jump, with the waist and midsection accentuated.

REPRISE: Do 8 basic jumps, swing the rope slowly side to side 16 times, and then 8 more basic jumps. That's your prelude to ...

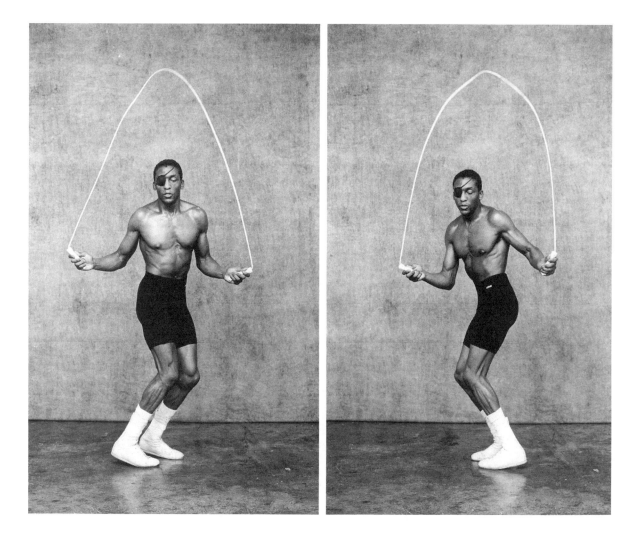

JUMPING JACKS

POSITION: Square off and grip the rope by its handles.

MOVEMENT: Football players do jumping jacks by swinging their arms so their hands meet at twelve o'clock, just above their heads. In this exercise, your feet mimic the traditional jumping jack, but you time your movements to the revolving rope. On the count of one, your feet extend laterally. On two, they come together. Out on three again. Back together on four. Continue until you've done 32 revolutions.

REMEMBER: Don't let your eyes deceive you. Although it seems impossible for your feet to go wide while the rope is turning, in actuality the rope will be behind and above your head, not down by your feet.

MUSCLES WORKED: The same muscles as in the basic jump, with the calves, lateral glutes, and soleus accentuated. This is a more explosive exercise than the previous ones.

REPRISE: Do 8 basic jumps, turn the rope side to side 16 times, then finish with another 8 basic jumps. That leads in to . . .

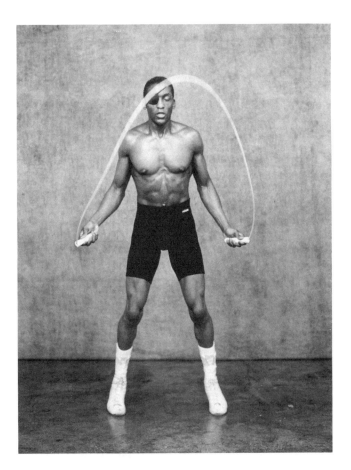

ANKLE CROSS JUMPS

POSITION: Square off and grip the handles of the rope.

MOVEMENT: As you jump, you simply cross your feet. On the count of one, the left foot crosses over the right, while the right foot crosses to the rear of the left. On two, you return to start position. On three, the right foot crosses over the left. Back to center on four. Continue until you've done 32 revolutions.

REMEMBER: One revolution of the rope per jump.

MUSCLES WORKED: The same muscles as in the basic jump, with the calves accentuated and your lower body agility and coordination tested.

REPRISE: Do 8 basic jumps, 16 figure eights, and 8 more basic jumps as a lead-in to the final rope exercise ...

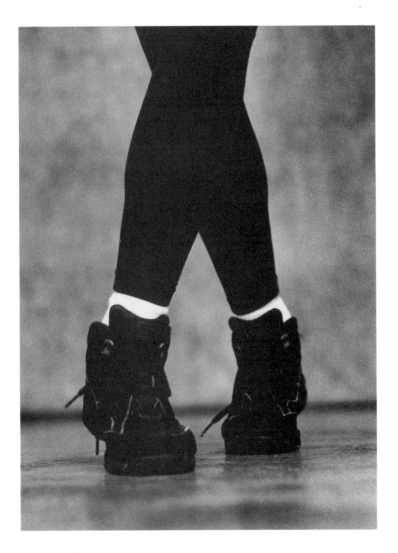

THE AEROBOX RUN

POSITION: Square off your stance and grip the rope by its handles.

MOVEMENT: As you turn the rope you kick your heels back, alternately, to simulate running. In fact, it's more like running in place. On the count of one, kick your right foot back as you turn the rope: on the count of two, kick your left foot back. Keep alternating until the count hits 16.

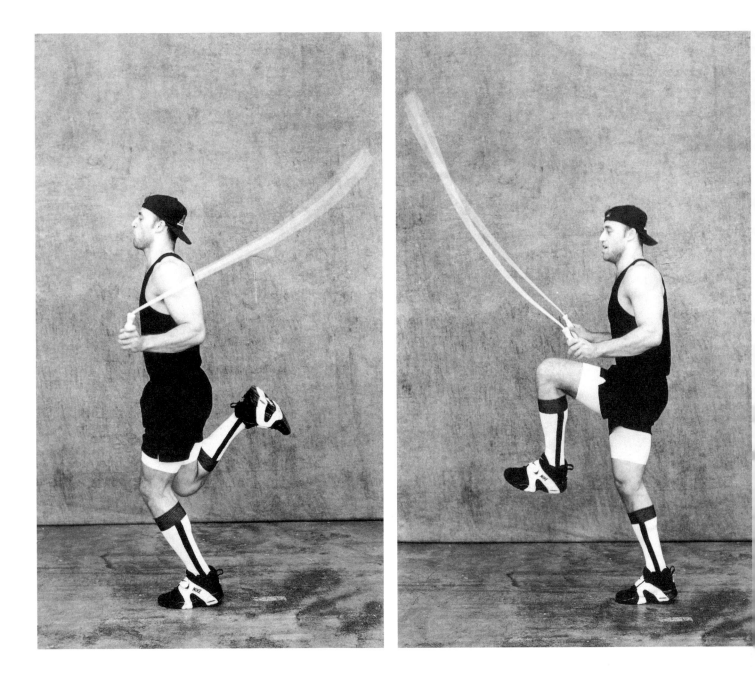

THE REST OF THE SEQUENCE: As you turn the rope, lift your knees exaggeratedly to simulate running. The movement resembles what football players do when they run tire drills. Right knee first (count of one), then left (count of two). Keep alternating until the count hits 16.

Then do the aerobic run for 8 revolutions of kicking your heels back and 8 more of lifting your knees. Repeat that two-part sequence for 4 revolutions each until you've done 32 revolutions in all. Repeat the sequence again, but this time for 2 revolutions of kicking your heels back and 2 of lifting your knees. Continue for 32 revolutions.

Then do 16 basic jumps and drop the rope.

MUSCLES WORKED: The same muscles as in the basic jump, with the hamstrings, glutes, and cardiovascular system accentuated. The abs are also emphasized because you are using them to help you lift your legs forward in the tire-drill jump.

This completes the rope segment of Aerobox. By now you should be huffing and puffing and thinking about the concept of mercy. If you're not fatigued, then you're a hardy specimen who's destined for the advanced workout sooner than most folks. For the rest of you, things get a bit easier in the next phase of Aerobox—body toning.

BODY TONING

OBJECTIVE: To bring down the heart rate from the intensity of the rope work . . . in preparation for a series of sit-ups and push-ups.

COOL-DOWN

SIDE STEPS

POSITION: Squared-off stance.

MOVEMENT: This exercise is performed at a normal walking pace. On the count of one, step laterally to the right with your right foot. On two, step laterally to the right with your left foot. On three, you move laterally to the left with your left foot. On four, laterally to the left with your right foot. Repeat for a total of 32 counts.

With these lateral steps your heart rate begins to return to normal.

OPTION: If your breathing is still very labored at this point, you may lengthen the count to 64, or simply walk back and forth until you begin to feel comfortable.

TWIST-AND-PUNCH

POSITION: Boxer's stance.

MOVEMENT: On the count of one, twist to the right and punch down with the left hand. On two, twist to the left and punch down with the right hand. Both the left and right hands are executed with a downward flicking motion. Repeat for 32 counts.

THE REST OF THE SEQUENCE: Repeat the same two-count twists, but this time elevate the punches to shoulder level for 32 counts. Then repeat the same two-count twists, and elevate alternate left and right hooks for a count of 32. Then, without the twists, alternate straight lefts and straight rights for a count of 32. The punches are thrown at a speed just above slow motion. This continues the process of restoring a normal heart rate, preparing you to do the ab workout on the floor.

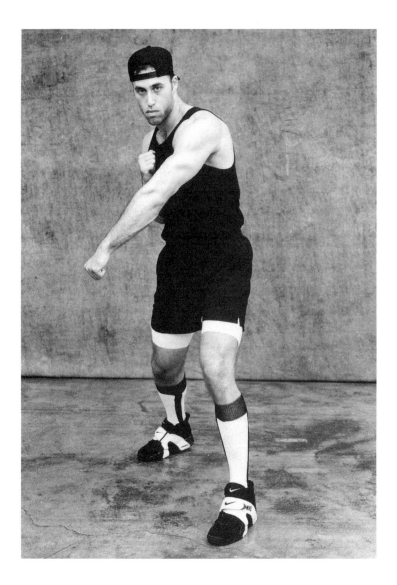

THE ABS

CRUNCHES

POSITION: You are in a sitting position, with your knees bent at 90 degrees. Your feet are flat to the ground, the toes are pointing straight ahead. Your fists are raised and in set position. Chin down and shoulders rolled. Abs tight. This will round you at your back and protect you from lower back strain.

MOVEMENT: Slowly lower down nine inches and raise up nine inches. As you come up, squeeze your abs and exhale lightly. As you go down, inhale through the nose. Up and back 8 times.

REMEMBER: These sit-ups, and the others you will perform, should be done in a controlled, tight arc. Your range of motion on the crunches is about nine inches forward and back.

OPTION: You may want to perform all sit-ups with a mat or thick towel under your body to reduce the severity of a hard floor.

MUSCLES WORKED: Upper abs.

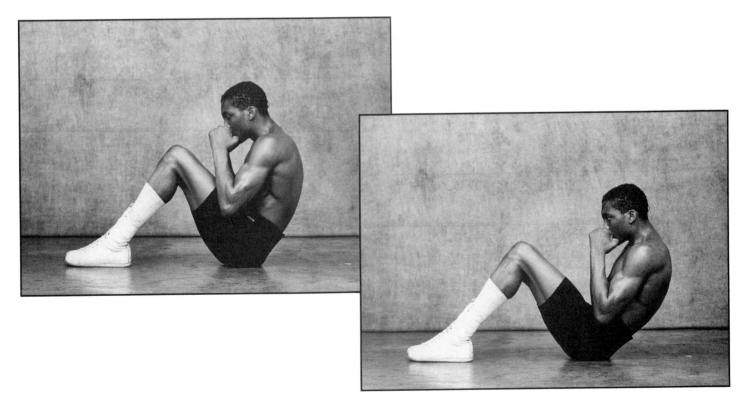

AEROBOX CRUNCH 'N' PUNCH

POSITION: Same as for crunches.

MOVEMENT: As you come up, thrust your left fist forward so that the elbow goes past the left knee. Keep the other fist in set position. Do that 8 times. With each crunch, your left fist comes back to set position. Then execute sit-ups in which you thrust your right fist forward so that the elbow goes past the right knee 8 times.

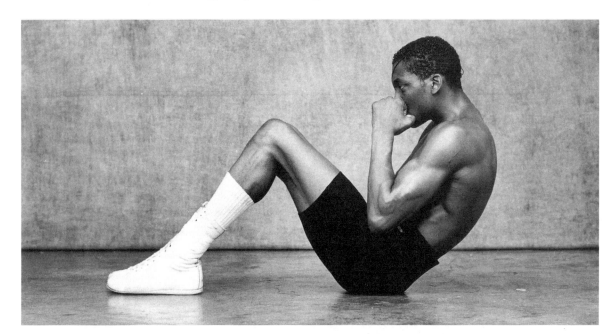

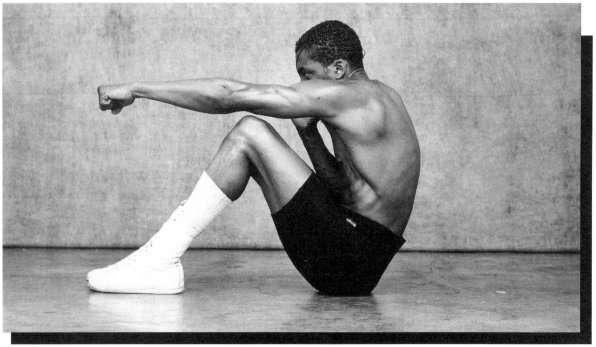

THE REST OF THE SEQUENCE: For the next set, with your hands in set position, tilt back to the maximum point in your nine-inch range of motion. At that point, twist to the left. As you rotate back to center, throw the left hook according to the techniques previously learned. Repeat 8 times.

Now do the same thing with the right hook, twisting to the right rather than the left. Repeat 8 times.

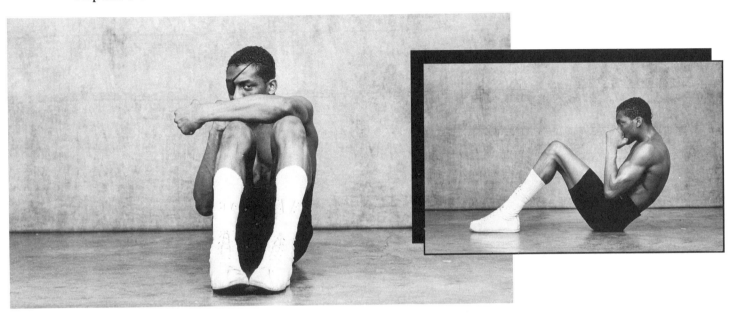

Next, twist to the left and deliver the left uppercut. Your left shoulder should be lower than your right shoulder as you punch and as you retract. When you twist to the left you are cocking your left shoulder. When the left shoulder swings forward, the left uppercut leaves the body. Throw the left uppercut eight times.

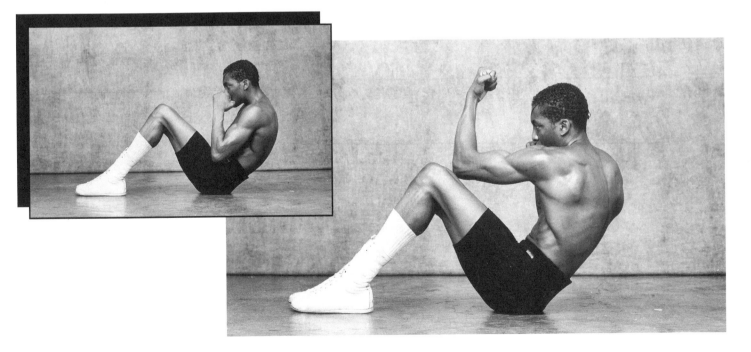

REMEMBER: In the initial crunch 'n' punch—where you thrust your fist forward—the other hand may grip the nether part of the thigh if you find that crunch, or any variation of the advanced crunches, hard to execute. It's a form of acceptable cheating that allows you to get some benefit from the exercise.

MUSCLES WORKED: Obliques and abs.

ELEVATED-LEG AB CRUNCHES

POSITION: You're on your back, with your legs elevated and bent 90 degrees at the knees. From the knees down your legs are somewhat parallel to the ground, but don't let your feet drop below your knees. Clasp your hands behind your head, which is about twelve inches off the ground.

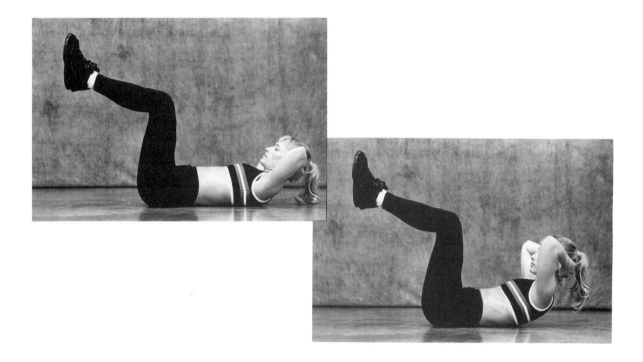

MOVEMENT: Using your shoulders and chest, lift up. It's a slow and controlled motion. Repeat 16 times.

REMEMBER: Don't tuck the elbows in. It limits your range of motion. And don't use your hands to jerk your head up. That's cheating and diminishes the benefits of this crunch.

MUSCLES WORKED: Upper abs.

ALTERNATING-LEG AB CRUNCHES

POSITION: You're on your back. Hands are clasped behind your head, which is twelve inches off the ground. Cross your left leg over the right thigh, just above the knee. The right leg is upraised at a 75-degree angle, toes pointing to the ceiling.

MOVEMENT: Rise up and guide your right elbow to your left knee, and then lower to set position. Repeat 8 times. Switch legs—right leg on top of upraised left—and touch your left elbow to the right knee.

THE REST OF THE SEQUENCE: Rotate to your left and touch your left knee with your right elbow for 4 counts, and then rotate to your right and touch your right knee with your left elbow for 4 counts. Do two 8-count sets. Then touch your right elbow to left knee twice, and left elbow to right knee twice, alternating until you've managed 8 sit-ups. Then alternate right elbow to left knee for one crunch and left elbow to right knee for one crunch until you've done 8 sit-ups.

VARIATION: If these crunches prove difficult for you, you can take the leg elevated at 75 degrees and drop your foot so it's flat against the floor.

MUSCLES WORKED: Abs and obliques.

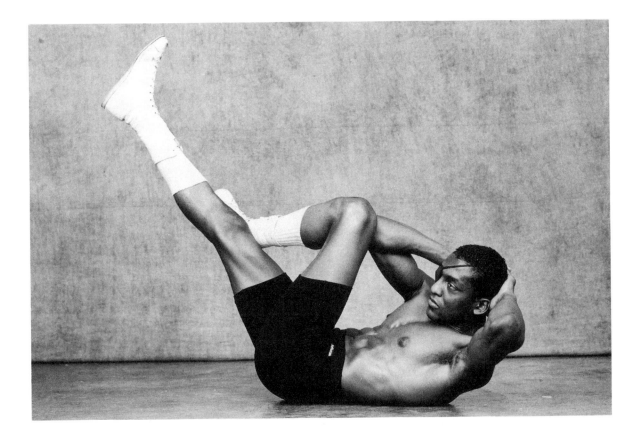

AB STRETCH

POSITION: Lie on your stomach with your arms extended in front of you. Toes point to the ground. Chin is up. The heels of your palms are on the ground, the fingers are pointing up. The thumbs may cross.

MOVEMENT: Raise your chest up as your hands slide back toward the body, and try to point your chin to the ceiling. Hold for a count of eight, inhaling as you come up. Exhale as you lower for a count of four, your hands returning to their original position. What stretches the abs is that pushing motion of your hands. Do 4 sets of upraises.

MUSCLES WORKED: Abs.

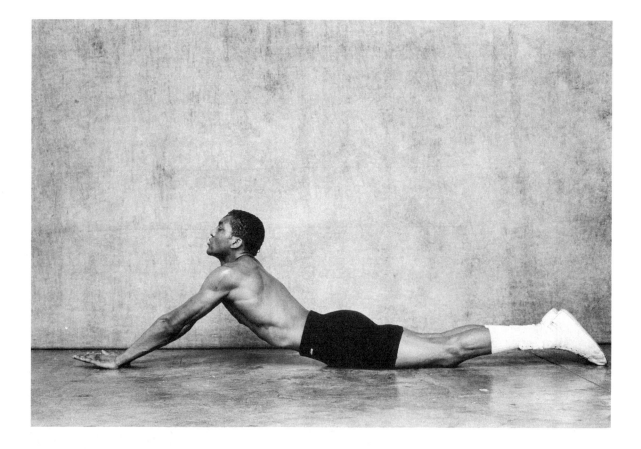

THUMBS-TOUCH PUSH-UPS

POSITION: Lie on your stomach, with your hands beneath your chest. Your fingers are flared, the sides of thumbs touching. The toes point to the ground.

MOVEMENT: Push yourself up and down in a controlled motion. Eight push-ups.

REMEMBER: Don't bounce when you come down. Brush your chest against your thumbs and then raise up. And don't let your elbows flare. Keep your back straight at all times.

OPTION: You can do these push-ups on your knees if they prove difficult from the prescribed position.

MUSCLES WORKED: Pecs, deltoids, and lats, with the back of the arms (triceps) accentuated.

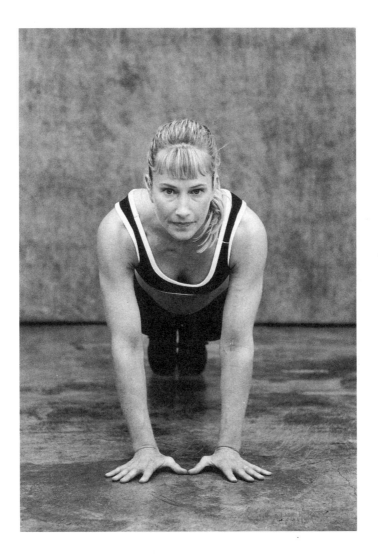

INVERTED PUSH-UPS

POSITION: You're on your hands and knees, your fingers facing in, your elbows flared out. Now elevate onto your toes, your weight on your hands. The degree of difficulty of these push-ups depends on how wide or tight you set your hands. When they are very wide or very tight, the inverted push-up is more difficult.

MOVEMENT: Slowly lower your body until your chest is an inch or two from the floor. Do 8 push-ups.

REMEMBER: Look straight ahead. Keep your buttocks raised up . . . to shoulder level. Don't let your back sag. When your back sags, you risk straining your back as well as diminishing the benefit of the push-up. As for the placement of your hands, the wider you make them the more your pecs have to work.

MUSCLES WORKED: Triceps, deltoids, lats, with the pecs accentuated.

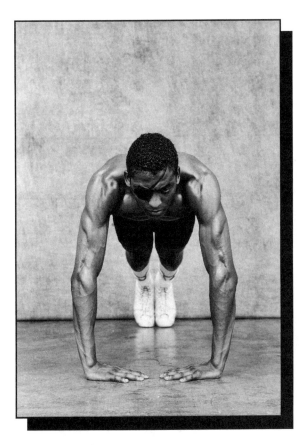

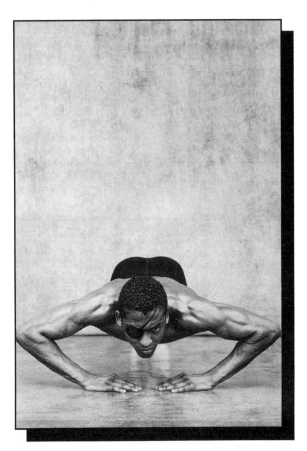

THRUST PUSH-UPS

POSITION: On your knees, put your hands about two feet out in front of you. The heels of the hands are touching the floor, with the palms and fingers raised. Straighten your legs so you're up on your toes.

MOVEMENT: Ease forward slowly, lowering only halfway down. To go further strains the elbow. Do 8 thrust push-ups with your hands shoulder-width apart and 8 with your hands set wider.

OPTION: For some of you, the thrust push-up may be beyond your present ability. An option is to perform the push-up on your knees.

MUSCLES WORKED: When your hands are shoulder-width apart, the emphasis is on the backs of the arms (triceps). The wider grip accentuates the lats. Also involved: the pecs and deltoids.

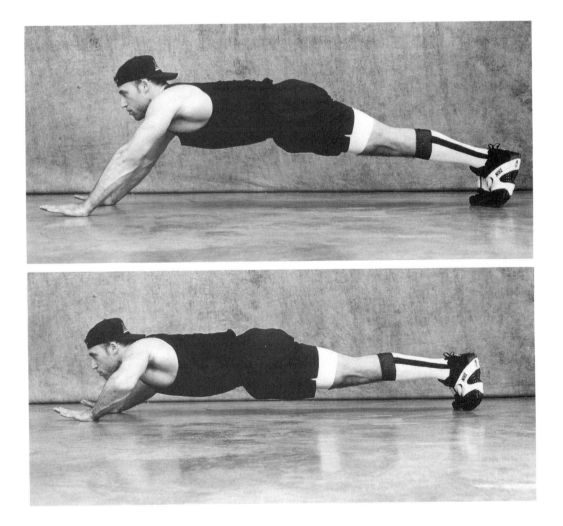

FINAL STRETCH AND COOL-DOWN

OBJECTIVE: To stretch the muscles of the upper and lower body to prevent soreness.

LAT STRETCH

POSITION: You're on your knees, with your feet tucked under you and your arms extended. The heels of your palms are pressed against the floor. Your head is bowed to the ground.

MOVEMENT: Stretch the arms forward, pull yourself back, and hold for 16 counts. This is a relaxation movement meant to bring your breathing under control.

REMEMBER: Don't sit back on your heels. You don't want to hurt your knees or ankles.

MUSCLES WORKED: The lats and the backs of your arms (triceps).

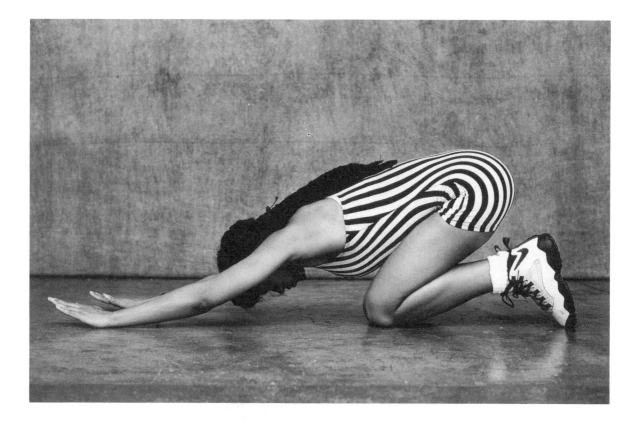

SHOULDER STRETCH

POSITION: On your knees, extend your right leg straight back and rise up on the toes of that foot. Your left hand is extended forward. The heel of the palm is flat against the ground. The right hand is flat against the floor, with the forearm vertical—as if in the push-up position.

MOVEMENT: Lean in to the right forearm and palm, pushing your chest lightly to the ground. Hold for eight to twelve seconds.

THE REST OF THE SEQUENCE: Take the left hand that was extended and place it under and across the chest so that your hand moves from twelve o'clock to three o'clock. The back of the hand is against the ground, with the palm up. The right forearm is ahead of the shoulder, and still in the push-up position. Lower your chest to the floor, pointing your nose downward. Hold for eight to twelve seconds.

Reverse sides and repeat both the movement and the rest of the sequence.

MUSCLES WORKED: For movement: lats and shoulder blade area. For rest of sequence: deltoids and upper shoulders.

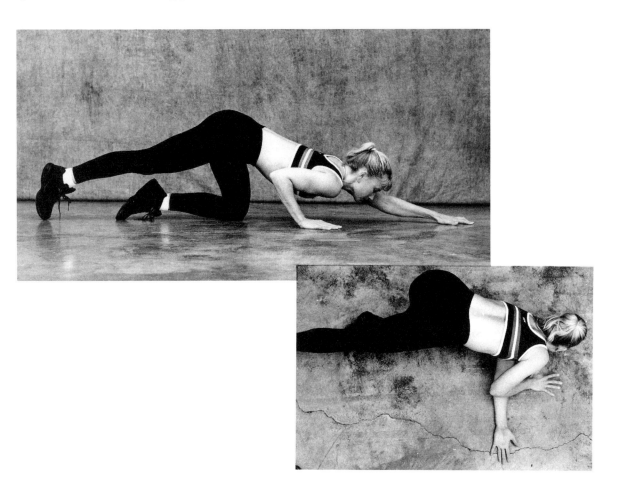

CALF STRETCH

POSITION: Your hands are under your chest and your torso is elevated and parallel to the ground. The left leg is extended and straight. Place your right foot on your left ankle. The ball of your left foot is flat against the ground, the heel is raised.

MOVEMENT: Push back with your hands, trying to get the left heel to move closer to the ground. Do this for a count of 12. Then reverse it so that the right calf is stretched.

MUSCLES WORKED: The calves.

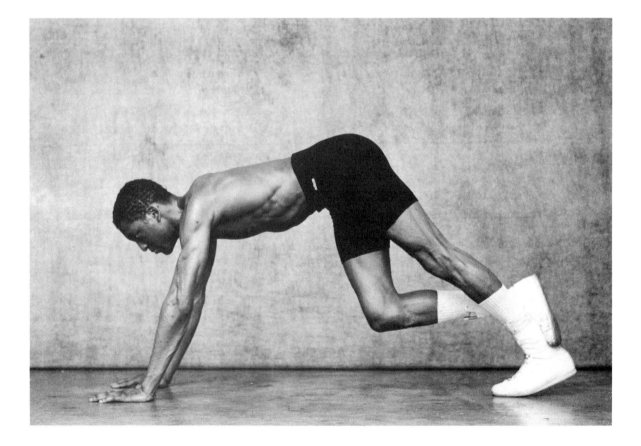

HAMSTRING STRETCH

POSITION: You're in a sitting position. Your legs are extended and flared—a V shape. Both hands grip your right ankle or lower legs.

MOVEMENT: Lean to your right knee and try to touch it with your forehead. Hold for a count of 12. With both hands, grip the left ankle and lean to your left knee, holding for a count of 12 again.

REMEMBER: Keep your legs straight. A lot of people will bend their knees and force the stretch. Don't force the stretch. The back of your knee is against the floor. Keep it that way when leaning to each side.

MUSCLES WORKED: Hamstrings.

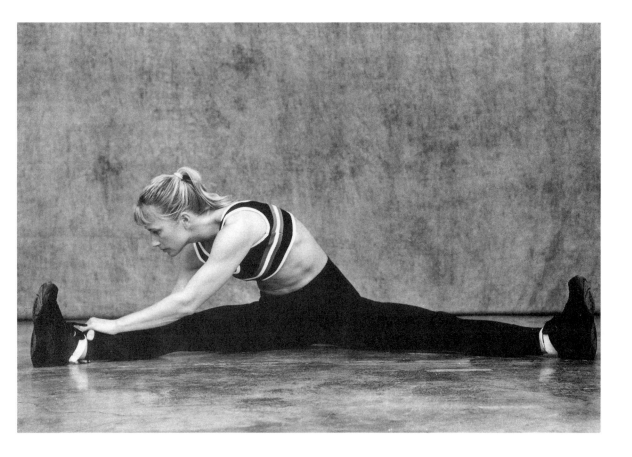

LOWER BACK STRETCH

POSITION: You are sitting with your left leg directly in front of you, toes pointing to the ceiling. Cross your right foot over your left knee so that it is flat to the ground. Your right hand is behind you, the palm against the ground and your fingers facing away from you. The triceps of your left arm rests against the outside of your right knee.

MOVEMENT: With your left arm, and as you look backward, push gently against the right knee for a count of 12. Then reverse legs and arms.

REMEMBER: If you have lower back problems, be very careful. Or bypass this stretch.

MUSCLES WORKED: Abs, obliques, and lower back.

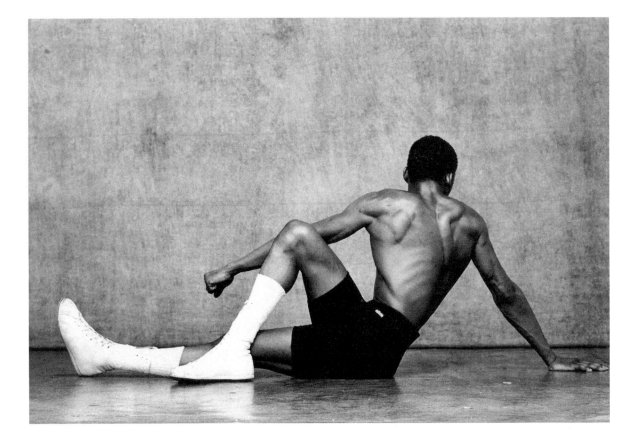

FIGURE FOUR STRETCH

POSITION: You're in a sitting position, with your right leg extended out in front of you. The bottom of your left foot is flat against the inner right thigh—a configuration that resembles the number four. Your right hand is holding your lower right leg, and your left hand is against the inside of the left knee.

MOVEMENT: Push down with the left hand against the inside of the knee as you lean to your right. Hold for a count of 12. Switch legs and hold for the same count.

REMEMBER: Don't bounce. You could irritate muscles if you do.

MUSCLES WORKED: Inner thighs and groin area.

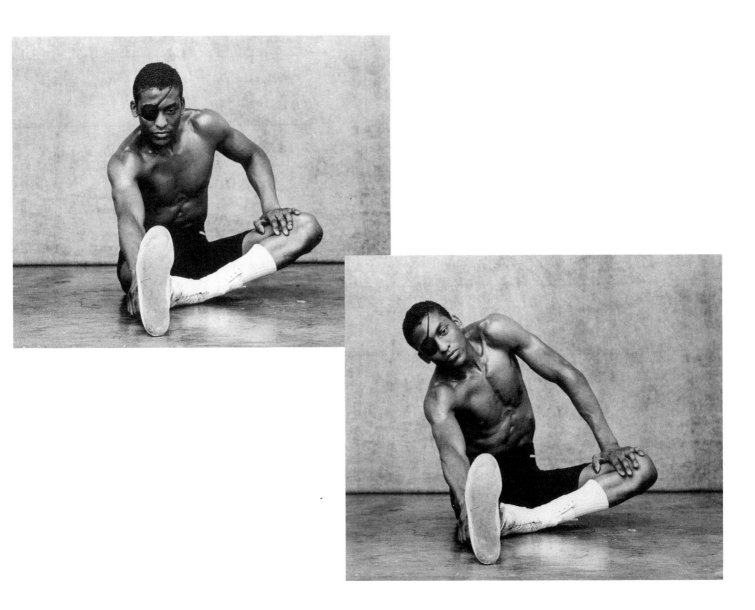

YOGA STRETCH

POSITION: You're in a sitting position, with the bottom of your feet touching and your legs flared. Your heels are as close as you can get them to your groin area. Clasp your hands and place them under your feet.

MOVEMENT: Push down toward the ground with the sides of your feet. Your back is straight and your chin is up so that you're looking toward the ceiling. Hold for a count of 8 and inhale.

THE REST OF THE SEQUENCE: As you pull yourself down, your chest and head lower toward your feet, and you exhale. Straighten your back and push down with your feet again. Hold for a count of 8.

MUSCLES WORKED: On the movement: traps. The rest of the sequence: the glutes.

This completes the beginner's Aerobox workout.

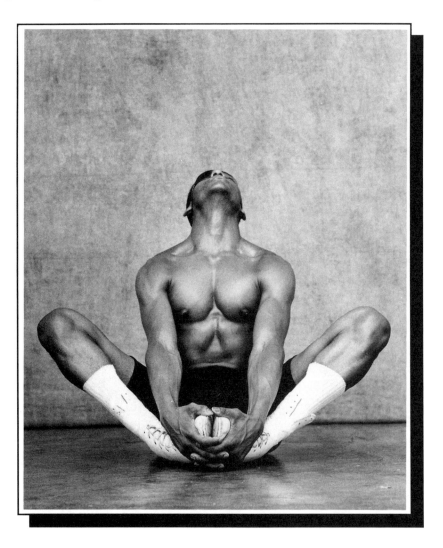

THE ADVANCED WORKOUT

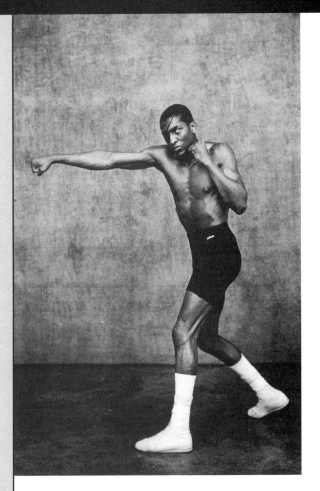

People differ in their eagerness to take on challenges.

Some folks are content to maintain the status quo, and feel no urgency about pushing their minds or bodies a dimension beyond.

In Aerobox, as in life, there are those for whom enough is enough—and those who want to test their developing skills.

If you're that go-getter sort, welcome to the advanced workout.

But even if you're not, I suggest you take a hard look at the particulars of the advanced program. Within it, you may find exercises to supplement your beginner's format. And who knows? That may pique your interest enough, eventually, to coax you to step up to the one-hour advanced workout.

If you're wondering what you're letting yourself in for by stepping up to the advanced workout, it's what you'd expect.

The workload is heavier, and

the exercises more demanding. For instance, the tricky technique of crossing the rope is part of the advanced workout. The push-ups tend to be more difficult—you won't easily execute the shovel push-up—and so are the sit-ups. The punching and skip-rope sequences are far more elaborate in this workout.

But if you've mastered the beginner's workout . . . if you no longer labor through that regimen . . . then very likely you have acquired the fitness necessary to tackle the rigors of advanced Aerobox.

BOXER'S SKIP
(without rope)

POSITION: Squared-off stance.

MOVEMENT: This is a movement that involves the subtle shift of weight from side to side. It is a bouncing, shifting movement that goes side to side on the balls of your feet. As you shift to the right, your right heel lowers to the ground without touching, and your left heel rises. Your weight also shifts to the right side. Then you shift to the left, repeating the same step on that side. This soft-shoe footwork is the basis of a fighter's most common method of skipping rope, but for this exercise you are without the rope. Do the boxer's skip for a count of 32. Your arms are at your sides. Your fists are closed.

THE REST OF THE SEQUENCE: Now, as you shift weight, add in a flicking punch downward to each side for 32 more counts. When you shift left, let the left hand go. When you shift right, it's the right hand you throw.

MUSCLES WORKED: Calves—and you're priming the rest of your body for the remainder of the one-hour advanced workout.

QUICK FEET

POSITION: Boxer's stance.

MOVEMENT: On the count of one, step forward with your left foot and bring your right foot forward. On two, step back with your right foot and then your left foot (see page 22). Continue for a total of 16 counts, executed slowly. Then do 64 counts at a rapid pace.

MUSCLES WORKED: Soleus, calves, and glutes.

REPRISED FROM BEGINNER'S WORKOUT: 1) 32 torso twists to the left and to the right (see pages 63–64); 2) 32 lateral slips, alternating left and right at a brisk pace (see page 24); 3) 32 V-slips to the left and right (see page 23).

ALI LEAN

POSITION: Boxer's stance, but with your hands down at your sides.

MOVEMENT: Drop your right foot back about nine inches and simultaneously twist your upper torso and face clockwise before returning to start position (see page 25). Do that slowly 8 times. Then drop your right foot back and twist your upper torso and face counterclockwise before returning to start position. Do that 8 times. Now do alternate twists clockwise and counterclockwise for a count of 32, executed at a somewhat more rapid pace. When you twist right or left, keep your eyes focused on the imagined opponent.

These movements mimic the unorthodox way Muhammad Ali had of eluding punches. The conventional wisdom is that a fighter should not lean back from punches—that he increases the likelihood of being hit when he does. Fighters are taught to avoid punches through lateral slips, V-slips, blocking, or by simply ducking. But of course Ali was no conventional fighter. He had superior reflexes that enabled him to get away with a move that would have been riskier for the average fighter. For you, this maneuver provides physical benefits while adding a bit of spice to the workout.

REMEMBER: When you step back, you want to tense your abs to relieve strain on your lower back. Make sure you don't pull so far back that your head and upper body go past your back foot.

MUSCLES WORKED: Obliques, calves.

THE TWIST-AND-PUNCH SERIES

POSITION: Assume a boxer's stance.

MOVEMENT: 1) With hands in set position, twist left and then right 16 times. 2) Twist left and right, punching downward at each rotation, for 32 times. 3) Muting your twist, throw alternating straight lefts and rights 32 times. 4) Twist left and right 16 times. 5) Twist left and right, throwing a left hook as you rotate right. Do that 8 times. 6) Twist to your right and throw the left hook. Twist to the left and throw the straight right. Do that 32 times. 7) Twist left and right 16 times. 8) Twist left and right and, as you rotate right, throw the left uppercut. Do that 8 times. 9) Twist right and then left, throwing the left uppercut as you rotate right and then the right hand as you rotate left. Do that 8 times. Remember to keep your left shoulder lower than your right when you throw that left uppercut. It's almost as though your body's tilted toward the left. 10) Twist left and right 16 times. 11) Twist left and right and, as you rotate left, throw the right uppercut 8 times. 12) Twist left and right, delivering the right uppercut as you rotate left and the left uppercut as you rotate right. For 32 punches in all. 13) Twist left and right 16 times. 14) Twist left and right and throw the right hook 8 times. 15) Twist left and right and throw the right hook and left hook 32 times. 16) Twist left and right 16 times. 17) Muting your twists, throw 32 alternating lefts and rights. 18) Finally, throw this combination of alternating straight punches: left-right, left-right-left, and right-left, right-left-right. Note: the three-punch portion is thrown at an accelerated speed, the three punches compressed into the same time span as the earlier two punches. The effect is like a rhythmic cha-cha-cha.

REMEMBER: For complicated punching sequences like this, you might want to reduce them to personal shorthand designations on scraps of paper that you can tape at eye level to a nearby wall or mirror in your workout area. That might make it easier to execute than having to keep glancing down at the book.

MUSCLES WORKED: Obliques, triceps, shoulder region, pecs.

REPRISE: 1) Shoulder stretch (hold for a count of 8). 2) Triceps stretch (hold for a count of 8). 3) Calf stretch (hold for a count of 10). 4) Hamstring stretch (hold for a count of 10). 5) Ankle looseners (hold for a count of 8).

This completes the opening warm-up and readies you for . . .

OPENING ROPE SEQUENCE

POSITION: Squared-off stance, gripping rope by the handles.

MOVEMENT: 1) Swing the rope side to side (count of one to the right, count of two to the left) slowly creating figure eights for 16 counts. 2) Side-to-side figure eights with calf raises every time you swing the rope to a side. For 32 counts. 3) Set your feet wide and do side-to-side figure eights for 8 counts, adding in a half squat every time the rope goes to the side. Do that for 32 half squats. 4) Bring your feet back to normal spacing and do 8 slow side-to-side figure eights, and then 8 side-to-side figure eights executed at a brisk pace. 5) Do 8 more side-to-side figure eights at a brisk pace and then 8 basic jumps. Continue the side-to-side figure eights and basic jumps until you've done 32 of each. 6) Do 32 more basic jumps. 7) Alternate one-footed hops, in groups of four, for 64 revolutions. 8) Sixteen basic jumps. 9) Alternate one-footed hops, in groups of two, for 32 revolutions. 10) Sixteen basic jumps. 11) Aerobox run, kicking your heels back, alternating left and right for 64 revolutions. 12) Sixteen slow side-to-side figure eights.

MUSCLES WORKED: Same as for basic jump, with calves, glutes, quads, and forearms accentuated.

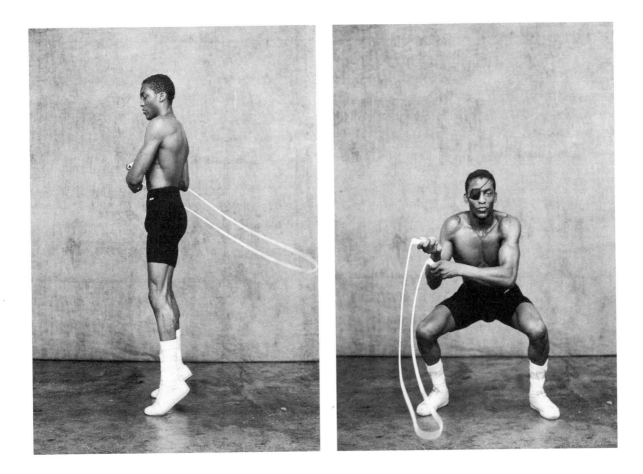

CROSSING THE ROPE

KEY ELEMENTS:

1. Your hands stay lower than your waist as you cross them over each other, and your forearms touch.
2. Your hands have to go wider than your body while crossed.
3. Maintain the jumping rhythm that preceded the maneuver.

POSITION: You're in a squared-off stance, holding the rope by the handles.

MOVEMENT: Do 8 basic jumps to get your rhythm. Then do 3 more basic jumps before your hands pass over each other, forearms touching (see page 33). By the numbers, it's basic jumps on the counts of one, two, three, cross on four. That four-count maneuver is one set. Do 16 sets.

REMEMBER: The mistake a lot of beginners make is to cut the crossing motion short. Rather than crossing the forearms and letting the hands swing wide of the body, they stop it before the arms cross, under the mistaken notion that the rope is going to catch at their feet. In actuality the rope is crossing behind them. Also, your hands must remain lower than your waist during the crossing over. If your hands are higher, you are in effect shortening the length of the rope, and your foot is more likely to snag the rope.

OPTION: If you're having trouble with this maneuver, lengthen the count. By the numbers, it's basic jumps on the counts of one, two, three, cross and hold on four and five, and basic jumps on six through eight. Holding for two beats usually forces individuals to visualize and feel the mechanics more readily and to turn the rope from the wrist, not from the arm.

MUSCLES WORKED: The same muscles as in the basic jump, with the pecs and shoulders accentuated.

REPRISE: Eight slow side-to-side figure eights as a lead-in to . . .

BOXER'S SKIP
(with rope)

POSITION: Squared-off stance, holding the rope by its handles.

MOVEMENT: As the rope turns, your right foot lands with the weight transferred and your left foot follows a quick beat later, the toes of that foot touching lightly against the floor and at a 45 degree angle. Then, on the next jump, the left foot plants and the right foot taps lightly against the floor. Do 32 revolutions. Then do a double boxer's skip. That means bouncing twice on the foot that plants. The other foot again taps gently and helps keep your balance. Do 32 revolutions.

THE REST OF THE SEQUENCE: Finish with 32 basic jumps.

MUSCLES WORKED: Same as in basic jump, with calves, soleus, foot, and ankle muscles accentuated. Because you constantly shift weight during this exercise, the stress on your calves is less than in the basic jump.

REPRISE: Do 8 slow side-to-side figure eights and put your rope down.

THE ADVANCED MULTI-PUNCH SERIES NO. 1

POSITION: Boxer's stance.

MOVEMENT: 1) Eight slow jabs; 2) 32 fast jabs; 3) 8 slow rights; 4) 32 fast rights; 5) 8 slow left hooks; 6) 3 rapid left hooks and rotate back to start position (16 sets); 7) 8 slow right uppercuts; 8) 32 rapid right uppercuts; 9) 8 slow left uppercuts; 10) 32 rapid left uppercuts.

MUSCLES WORKED: Upper and lower body muscles previously mentioned in punching exercises.

THE ADVANCED MULTI-PUNCH SERIES NO. 2

POSITION: Boxer's stance.

MOVEMENT: 1) Lateral slip to left and jab; 2) lateral slip to right and straight right hand; 3) V-slip to the left and left hook; 4) V-slip to the right and straight right hand; 5) 8 alternate lefts and rights. This sequence comprises a set. Do 8 sets with a four-second break between each set.

THE REST OF THE SEQUENCE: You perform this series at a rapid pace: 1) Lateral slips left and right, executed as quickly as you'd deliver a double jab. 2) V-slips left and right. 3) Alternate quick jab, right hand, jab, right hand. 4) As you back up (right foot back first, then left), you jab off the second step. Then repeat this movement, finishing with another jab. Repeat this sequence, numbers one to four, 8 times.

MUSCLES WORKED: Upper and lower body muscles previously mentioned in punching and slipping exercises.

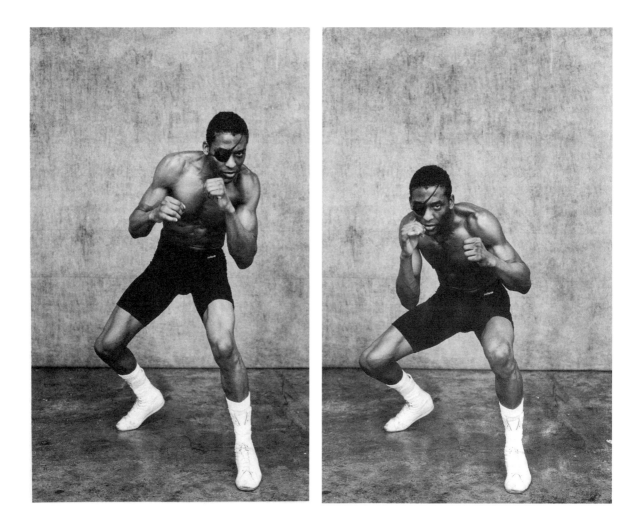

THE OLAJIDÉ SPECIAL COMBINATION SERIES

POSITION: Boxer's stance.

MOVEMENT: Series No. 1 includes steps one to six. 1) Zigzag ducking movement left and right (lowering from the knees and executed at the speed of a double jab) and then throw the right uppercut; 2) right, left hook, right; 3) lateral slip left and right, followed by a right uppercut; 4) right, double left hook, and right, simultaneously taking two steps forward, moving hard and somewhat crouched, twisting slightly to the left on the first step and slightly to the right on the second step; 5) then as you plant your feet, throw a right uppercut, straight right, left hook and right, moving a simple step forward with each punch; 6) then back to the twisting zigzag maneuver, followed by a right, double left hook, and right, moving a simple step forward with each punch. Series No. 2 includes steps seven to thirteen: 7) Duck (bending from the knees) and twist to the right—do the sequence 4 times; 8) duck, twist to right, and add a straight right—do the sequence 4 times; 9) duck, straight right, and add in a left hook—4 times; 10) duck, straight right, and double left hook—4 times; 11) duck, straight right, double left hook, and right again—4 times; 12) duck, straight right, double left hook, right, and left uppercut—4 times; 13) duck, then moving a step forward with each punch, execute a straight right, double left hook, right and left uppercut.

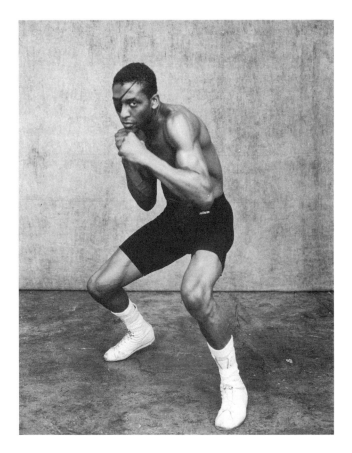

NEXT PHASE: 1) Duck and bounce on your toes, counting to eight; 2) duck and step forward, then throw your right, twisting your body into it; retreat to start position; do the sequence 4 times; 3) duck and step forward, throw your right and left hook before returning to start position; do this movement 4 times; 4) duck, right hand, left hook, and another right; return to start position; do the sequence 4 times; 5) duck, right-left-right and add another left hook; do that sequence 4 times; return to set position; 6) add a straight right hand and do that sequence 4 times; 7) add a left hook and do the sequence 4 times, but pause after the first three punches of the sequence so your combination will be duck, right-left-right, pause, left-right-left; return to set position.

MUSCLES WORKED: Upper and lower body muscles previously mentioned in punching and slipping exercises.

The Olajidé Special Combination Series completes this punching phase and segues to ...

ADVANCED RAPID-ROPE SERIES

POSITION: Squared-off stance, gripping the rope by the handles.

MOVEMENT: 1) Side-to-side figure eights, 32 times; 2) 64 basic jumps; 3) crossovers on the first of every 8 revolutions (basic jumps in between) for 64 revolutions; 4) crossovers on the first of every 4 revolutions ... for 32 revolutions (basic jumps in between); 5) crossovers on the first and second revolutions of every 8 revolutions ... for 64 revolutions (basic jumps in between); 6) 16 basic jumps; 7) 32 boxer's skips; 8) 16 side-to-side figure eights; 9) 16 revolutions of Aerobox run; 10) 16 revolutions of tire drill; 11) 8 revolutions of Aerobox run; 12) 8 revolutions of tire drill; 13) 2 revolutions of Aerobox run; 14) 2 revolutions of tire drill; 15) 16 basic jumps; 16) 8 slow side-to-side figure eights; 17) 16 basic jumps.

MUSCLES WORKED: Same as for the basic jump, with the pecs, abs, gastrocnemius, hamstrings, and calves accentuated and the cardiovascular system severely tested.

SPEED SKATING

POSITION: Squared-off stance, gripping rope by handles.

MOVEMENT: Lean forward, as a speed skater does. As you jump, kick your left heel back so that it crosses at the rear of the right leg. That's count of one. On two, kick your right heel back so that it crosses at the rear of the left leg. Continue for 64 nonstop revolutions of the rope.

REMEMBER: This is similar to the Aerobox run rope exercise. But in the Aerobox run, you kick your heel straight back. In speed skating you turn the heel so that it bisects the leg at the back of the knee. At that moment, the toes of your raised foot will be pointing down. That straight leg will be slightly wide of your shoulder.

I began doing this exercise in the gym after seeing old film clips of U.S. speed skater and multi-gold-medalist Eric Heiden in the Olympics.

MUSCLES WORKED: Same as the basic jump, with the quads and hamstrings accentuated.

REPRISE: Sixteen side-to-side figure eights and 16 basic jumps as a lead-in to . . .

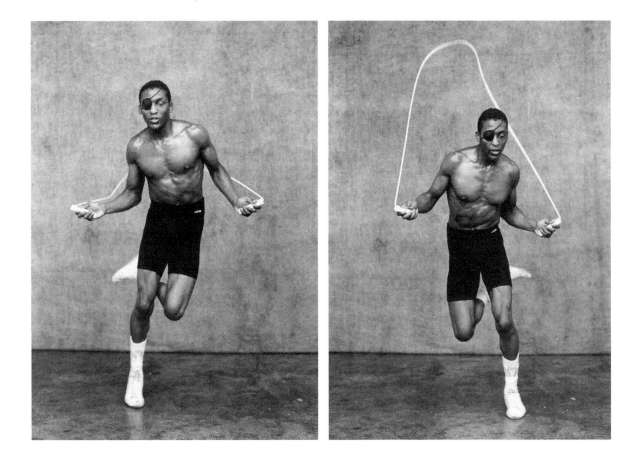

THE ABBREVIATED 911

POSITION: Squared-off stance, holding rope by the handles.

MOVEMENT: In this exercise, you do the tire-drill knee raises for two counts, alternating left then right, then accelerate the movement for counts three-four-five. That five-count movement is one set. Do 8 sets.

REMEMBER: The rope speeds up on the accelerated beats. You must get your knees high as you jump. Those accelerated beats I refer to as the "emergency run." That's how the "911" got to be incorporated into the name of the exercise. It has the cha-cha-cha syncopation you experienced in the twist-and-punch series.

MUSCLES WORKED: Same as the basic jump, with the glutes, abs, and calves accentuated.

REPRISE: Sixteen side-to-side figure eights as a lead-in to . . .

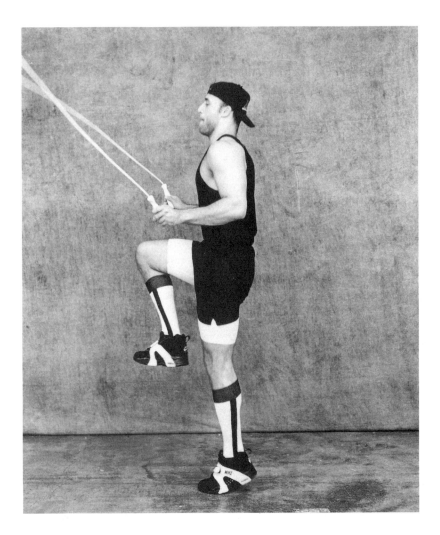

DOUBLE JUMPS AND MORE RAPID ROPE

POSITION: Squared-off stance, gripping rope by the handles.

MOVEMENT: Begin with seven basic jumps. As you get to the eighth jump, you must leap higher and turn the rope twice before your feet touch the ground (see page 36). Do that for 64 jumps, with your double turn of the rope coming on every eighth beat.

THE REST OF THE SEQUENCE: Double up on every fourth beat for 64 more revolutions of the rope. Then do 16 side-to-side figure eights, and 16 basic jumps. Do a single side-to-side as fast as a double jab, followed by 7 basic jumps, and continue for a total of 32 counts. Then an accelerated side-to-side, followed by 7 basic jumps for a total of 64 counts. Finally, an accelerated side-to-side, followed by 3 basic jumps for a total of 32 counts.

REMEMBER: The lift on the big jumps comes from the calves. Keep your weight centered. Don't tilt back. If you do, you'll lose your balance and fall backward.

MUSCLES WORKED: Same as for the basic jump, with the calves, soleus, shoulder region, forearms, biceps, and pecs accentuated.

REPRISE: Sixteen side-to-side figure eights and 16 basic jumps as a lead-in to . . .

ANKLE TOUCHES

POSITION: Squared-off stance, gripping the rope by the handles.

MOVEMENT: With your feet shoulder-width apart, as you jump, bring your feet together so that the ankles touch in midair on the count of one. On counts two through eight, do basic jumps. Continue for 64 counts.

THE REST OF THE SEQUENCE: Ankles touch on counts one and two, basic jumps on three through eight. Continue for 32 counts. Ankles touch on counts one through three. Basic jumps four through eight. Continue for 32 counts. Ankles touch counts one through four, basic jumps five through eight. Continue for 32 beats. Then 32 consecutive revolutions of the rope in which your ankles touch on every turn. Finish with 16 basic jumps and 16 slow side-to-side figure eights. Put the rope down.

REMEMBER: Don't let your feet come out too wide.

MUSCLES WORKED: Same as for the basic jump, with the calves and soleus accentuated.

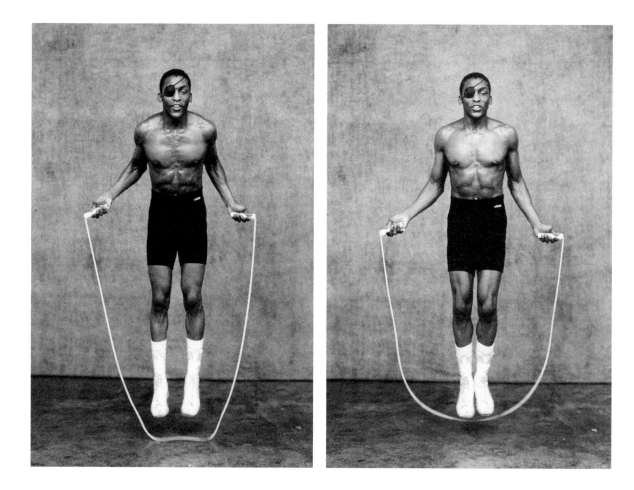

FEINT AND FIRE

POSITION: Boxer's stance.

MOVEMENT: Move aggressively two steps forward and feint with your head by moving your head quickly from left to right. Do that step and feint 8 times.

REST OF SEQUENCE: Repeat your two-steps-and-feint maneuver, then spring back one step. That's one set. Do 8 sets. Then, as you retreat, add a left hook. Do 8 sets. To the left hook, add a right hand. Eight sets. To the left hook, right, add a left uppercut. Eight sets.

REMEMBER: When you step forward, you're sliding on the front of your foot.

MUSCLES WORKED: All the muscles as previously indicated from the various punches, with the calves and quads accentuated.

REPRISE: 1) Sixteen side-to-side steps; 2) 32 shoulder shrugs, rolling the shoulders forward; 3) 32 shoulder shrugs, rolling the shoulders backward.

NECK NODS

POSITION: You're on your back, with your legs bent at the knee, feet flat against the floor. Your arms are naturally at your sides. Your head and shoulders are off the ground.

MOVEMENT: Slowly roll your neck forward, and back, over a six-inch arc. Your objective is to touch your chin to your chest. It's a nodding movement, as though you're nodding yes, and it is executed economically. Go up and back 64 times.

REMEMBER: After you rotate your neck forward, be sure to control the reverse movement. Don't just drop your head down. Keep your teeth clenched as you roll forward and back.

MUSCLES WORKED: Neck and face muscles.

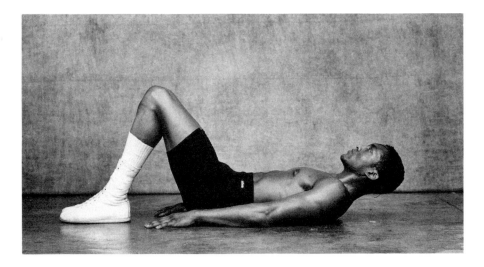

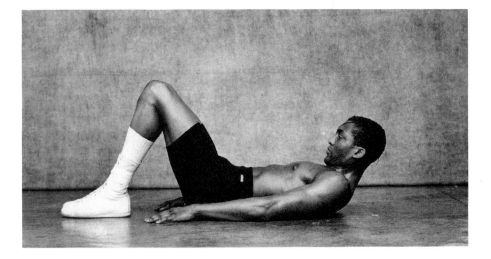

TWISTING AB CRUNCHES

POSITION: You're on your back, hands clasped behind your head. Your legs are elevated and bent at the knee. From the knees down, your legs are roughly parallel to the floor.

MOVEMENT: On the count of one, lift up and then twist your right shoulder to the left knee, then back to center on two. On three, rise up again and twist your left shoulder to the right knee. Return to start position on four. That constitutes one set. Do 16 sets.

MUSCLES WORKED: Abs and obliques.

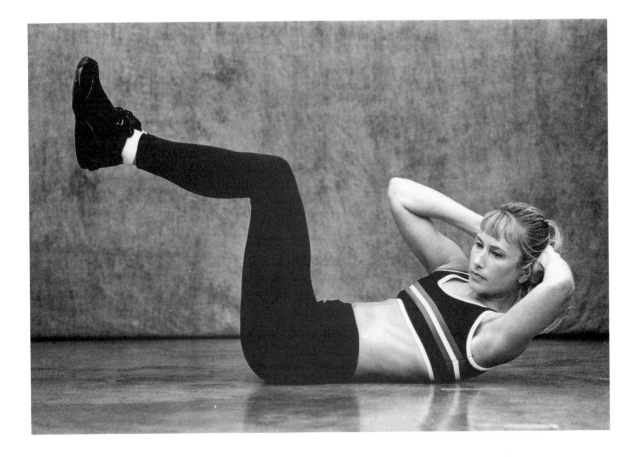

SWIVEL LEG EXTENSIONS

POSITION: Same as for twisting ab crunches.

MOVEMENT: Do 16 double-leg extensions: the legs extend outward and then return to start position. Without pause, and with your feet together, swivel the hips to the right, and then back to the left. Do that 32 times at a moderately paced speed. Then 32 more at an accelerated speed. Then repeat at both speeds, swiveling to the left and the right. The movement has a resemblance to break dancing.

REMEMBER: When you swivel right, you should see the outside of your right foot. Swiveling left, you'll see the outside of your left foot. Keep your head and shoulders off the ground so the lower back stays pressed to the floor. Do not move the upper body as you swivel.

OPTION: To make the exercise easier, you may place your fists beneath your buttocks rather than clasping your hands behind your head.

MUSCLES WORKED: Mostly the obliques.

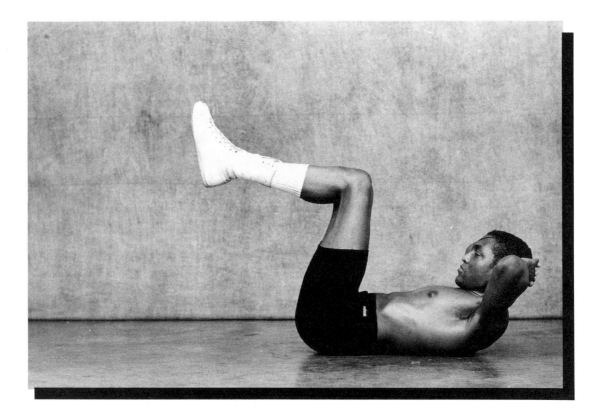

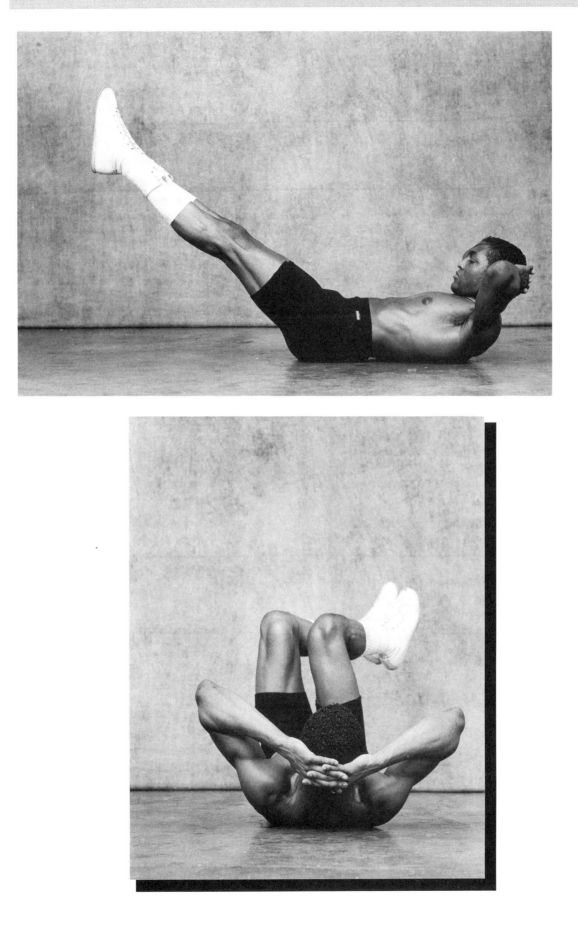

V-SITS

POSITION: You're on your back, legs extended and parallel to the ground. Your hands are at your sides. Your abs are tensed.

MOVEMENT: Take a deep breath through your nose and, as you hold your breath, raise your legs (with ankles touching) off the ground. Keep them straight as you bring your upper body off the floor. From a side view, your body looks like a V, which explains the name of this exercise. Hold that V position for a count of eight and then lower slowly for a count of eight, keeping your legs about twelve inches off the ground and your upper torso about the same. As you lower your legs, your breathing is shallow. Throughout the exercise, your lower and upper body simultaneously rise up and down, and your buttocks stay clenched. Do 4 sets of eight beats up and eight beats down.

REMEMBER: In this type of sit-up, you need to be aware of the muscles you're working. Some people cheat by not keeping their legs straight, which diminishes the benefits you get by doing the V-sit properly. If you find yourself inclined to cheat, here's a suggestion: keep your fingertips on the ground.

OPTION: If these V-sits are too hard on your back, then lower your legs, bending at the knee.

MUSCLES WORKED: Abs.

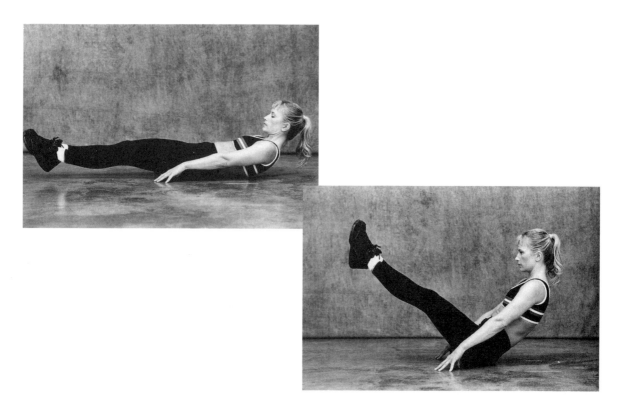

LATERAL V-SITS

POSITION: You're on your side, leaning on your left forearm, which is flat to the ground, the fingers pointing straight ahead. The right arm is extended across the body, the fingertips cupped and touching the floor.

MOVEMENT: Raise both legs laterally and straight up off the ground. As you do that, your upper torso swings forward with the motion. Raise the legs up and down 16 times. Then switch sides and do 16 more lateral V-sits. Repeat from both sides, but this time for only 8.

OPTION: To make the lateral V-sit easier, you can just lift the upper leg while holding the bottom leg four to six inches off the ground.

MUSCLES WORKED: Obliques, lateral thighs, and glutes.

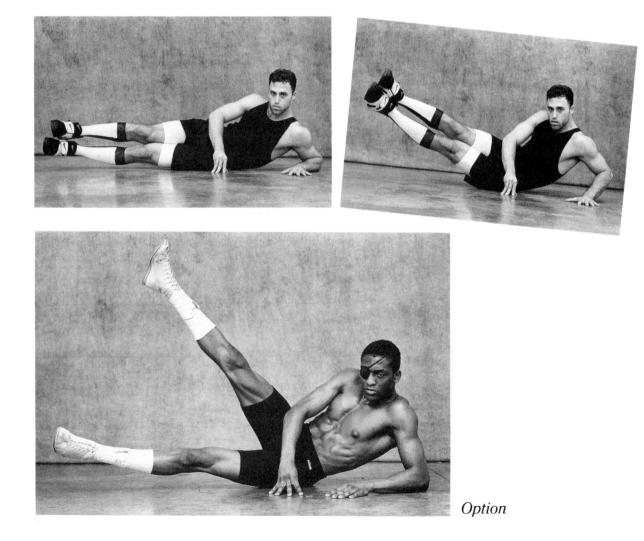

Option

TWISTING OBLIQUE STRETCH

POSITION: You're on your back, your arms extended over your head, your hands clasped, and your legs straight.

MOVEMENT: Take a deep breath and then lean from the shoulders, to the left first (hold for eight) and then lean to the right (hold for eight). Keep your upper back pressed firmly against and sliding along the floor. Do 2 sets like that.

THE REST OF THE SEQUENCE: The ab stretch from the beginner's workout (see page 94).

MUSCLES WORKED: Obliques.

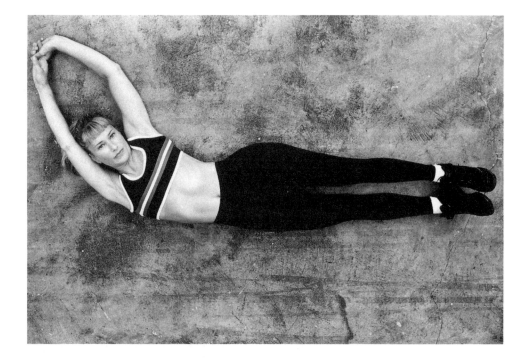

INVERTED TRICEPS PUSH-UPS

POSITION: On your knees. Your hands are in an inverted position, the right hand ahead of the left, the right thumb touching the left pinky.

MOVEMENT: Rise up on your toes and lower down eight times. Your legs should be spread apart. Take a twenty-second break and do 8 more inverted triceps push-ups.

OPTIONS: If you find these push-ups difficult, you can try them on your knees, with your knees together (the easiest way), or with your knees spread apart.

MUSCLES WORKED: Pecs, triceps.

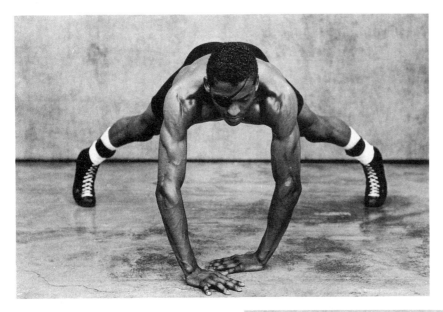

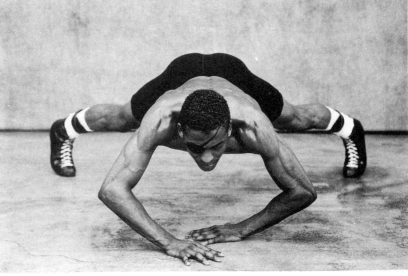

SHOVEL PUSH-UPS

POSITION: Your right hand is under your chest. The left hand is extended about two feet out in front of your shoulders, the fingers pointing forward. Your right leg is extended behind you, the toes gripping the ground. Your left leg is bent at the knee, with the foot pointing up.

MOVEMENT: Look to your left and then roll slightly in that direction—a kind of cocking movement. Then uncock by a slow swooping motion downward. That cocking and uncocking gives the push-up a kind of shoveling effect. Do that 8 times. Then switch sides and do 8 more shovel push-ups, looking to your right. Once completed, take a twenty-second break.

OPTION: This is a difficult push-up. One way to make it easier is to do it from one knee.

MUSCLES WORKED: Pecs, lats, deltoids, upper triceps, and shoulders.

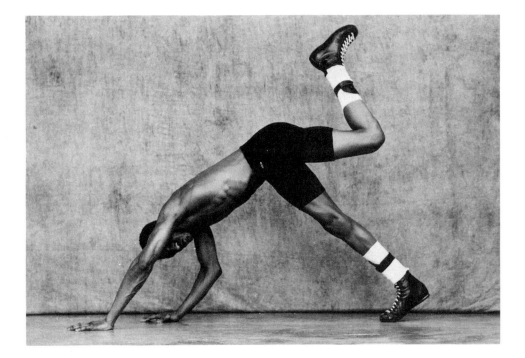

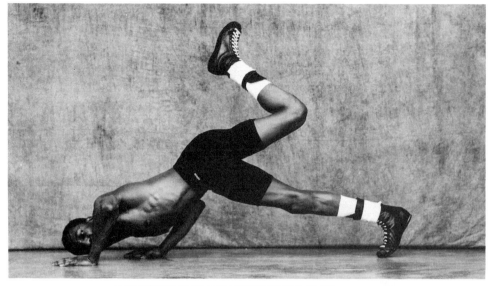

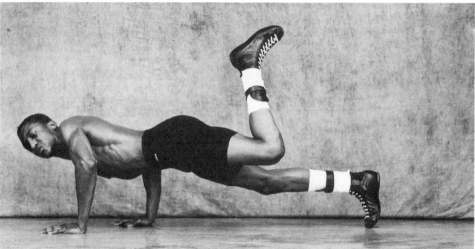

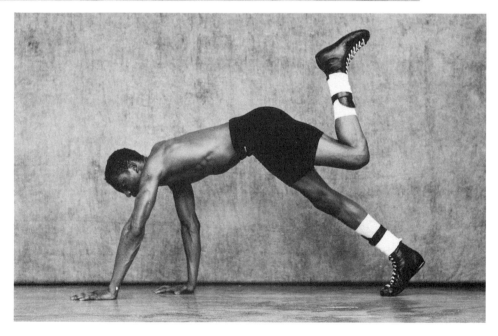

DOUBLE-BOUNCE PUSH-UPS

POSITION: You're on your toes in the push-up position, hands under your shoulders.

MOVEMENT: Lower your body with a controlled motion. Brush your chest against the floor and come partway up before lowering again and then elevating to start position. This is a pumplike motion. On the second of this two-part push-up, it is as though you free-fall toward the ground and catch yourself before hitting, and then you push your body back up. This push-up should be performed more rapidly than the basic push-up. Do 8 double-bounce push-ups, take a twenty-second break, and do 8 more.

OPTION: If these push-ups are difficult for you, you may do them on your knees.

MUSCLES WORKED: Biceps, pecs, triceps, and shoulders.

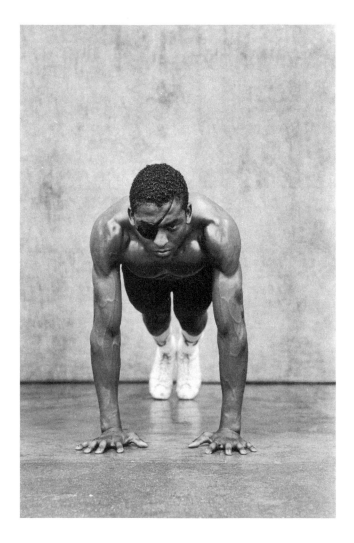

TRICEPS SITS

POSITION: You're in an elevated sitting position. Your hands are at your sides, palms down, supporting your weight. Your butt is about nine inches off the ground. Your fingers point straight ahead.

MOVEMENT: Lower yourself, bending the elbows, for eight triceps sits. Then follow with a set of 8 double-bounce triceps sits. Take a twenty-second break and repeat both sets.

MUSCLES WORKED: Triceps and delts.

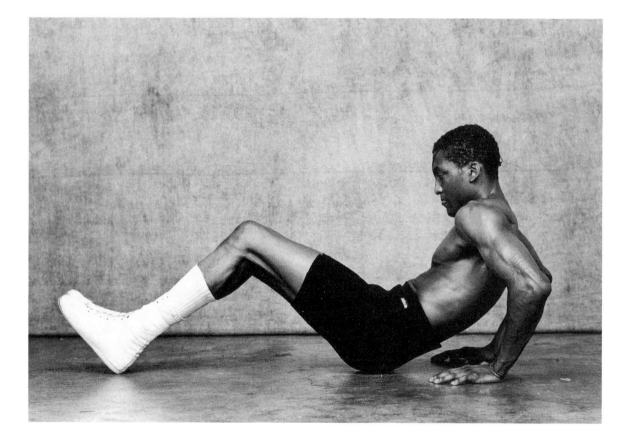

SITTING SERIES STRETCH

POSITION: You are seated, with your left foot touching the inner right thigh, by the knee.

MOVEMENT: Reach forward for your extended lower right leg or ankle. As you come forward, touch your head to your right knee and hold for a count of eight. Rise up for a count of four. Lower for eight. Up for four. This exercise stretches the hamstrings.

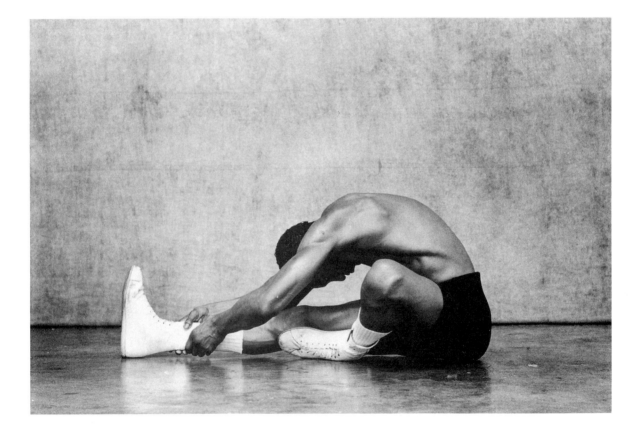

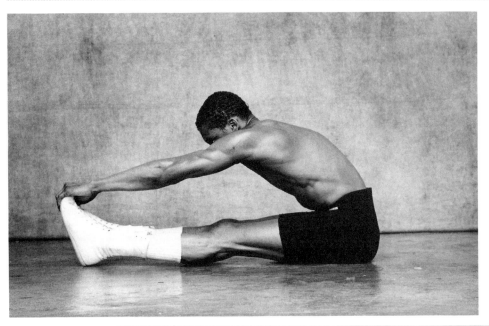

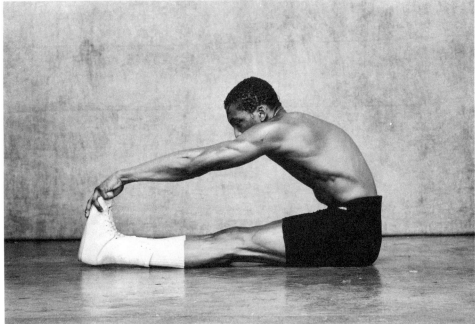

THE REST OF THE SEQUENCE: 1) Place your left hand on the bent left knee, your right hand on the extended right leg, by the ankle. As you lean to the right, push down on your left knee for a count of eight. This stretches the hips, inner thighs, and obliques. Come back to the center and relax for a count of four. Then repeat the twelve-count set. Then switch legs and repeat.

2) Now sit with both legs straight and extended out in front of you. Grip your toes. Push your toes forward for a count of eight, stretching the lats and triceps. Then grab your feet and pull toward you for eight, watching your heel rise up off the ground. This stretches your calves. Those two parts comprise one set. Do 8 sets.

3) You're still in a sitting position. Both legs are bent and set wide, feet flat to the floor. Your palms are together, your ring finger and pinky are pointed toward and are touching the ground. The triceps of each arm is against the inner thigh of each leg, just above the knee. Inhale through the nose and, as you lean forward, simultaneously push in with the knees, chin down, and then release by letting your legs flair wide. As you push, hold for a count of four. As you release, you merely relax for a count of eight. Do that 4 times to stretch the upper back muscles and triceps.

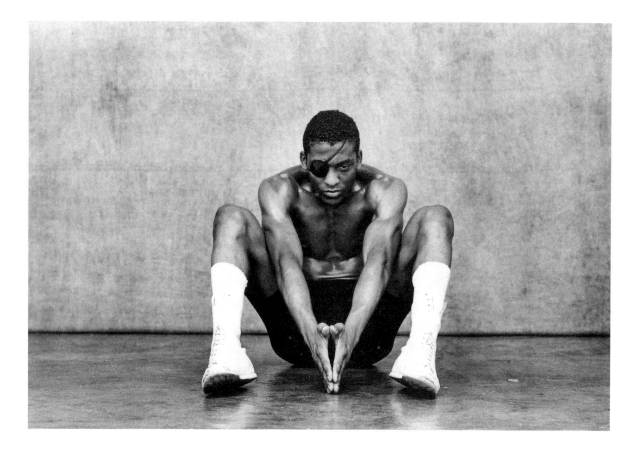

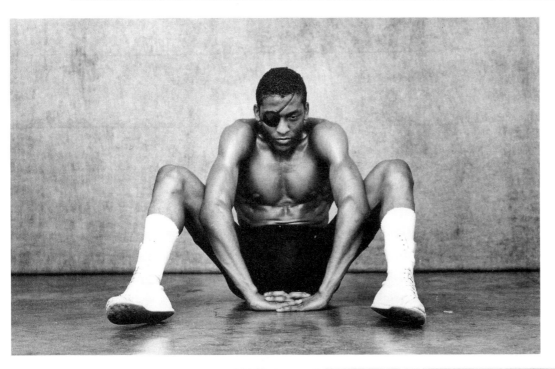

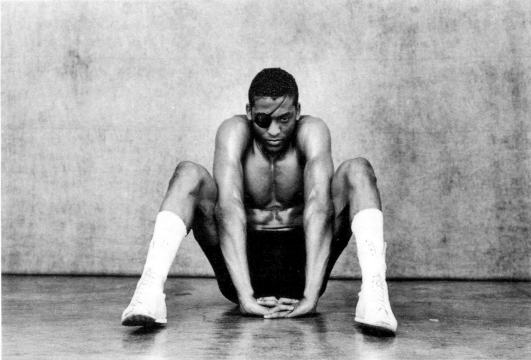

4) You are still seated, with your elbows against the insides of your legs, just above the knees, and your hands interlocked. Place those interlocked hands flat to the ground, then push in with your knees so the elbows almost look like they're pointing forward. Hold for a count of eight. Release for a count of four. The stretch is in the rear deltoids and the shoulder. Do that 4 times.

5) Switch to a kneeling position, with both legs under you, and do the shoulder stretch (see page 67) from the beginner's workout, using a count of eight for each shoulder.

6) Finally, extend your right leg, which is to the rear. With your left leg forward, lean forward to stretch the hip flexors and hold for a count of eight. Then relax for a count of eight. That's one set. Do 4 sets. Then switch legs and repeat.

This completes the one-hour advanced Aerobox workout.

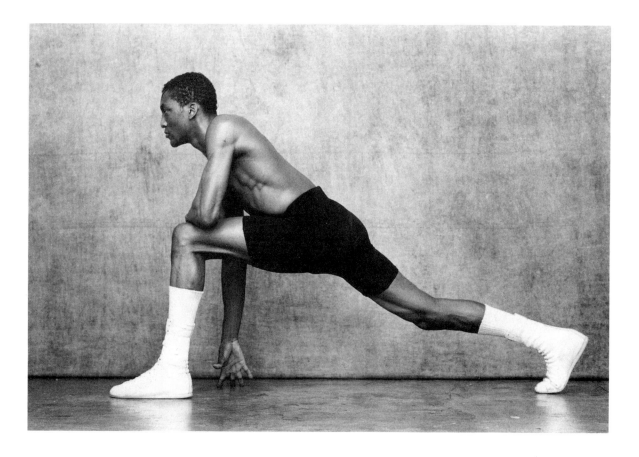

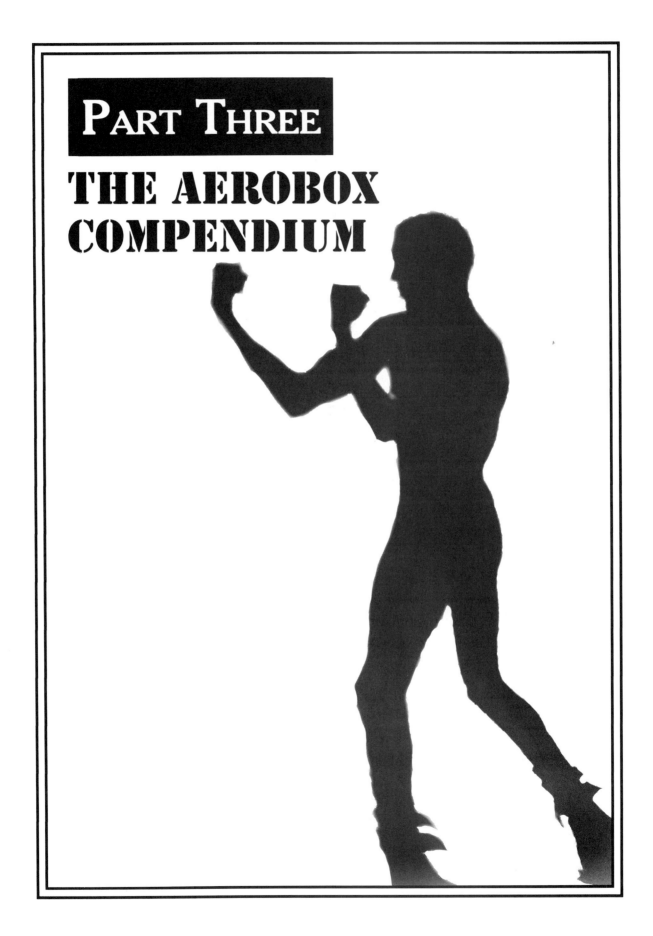

PART THREE

THE AEROBOX COMPENDIUM

Aerobox started from a simple impulse: a way for me to stay fit.

But in a few short years, it's gone far beyond that, becoming an enterprise that now exists against a more complicated backdrop—a world of commercial, social, psychological, even sexual nuance.

This book was conceived as a primer that would give you the broad strokes of a new exercise format and then lay out detailed specifics on how to do it.

By that game plan, there were many tangents that, though interesting, simply didn't belong up front of the book.

So . . . Part Three is the repository of those tangential matters—an odd lot of thoughts, perceptions, and advice that, with any luck, may inform and entertain you.

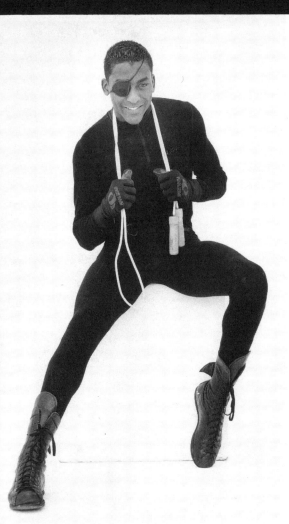

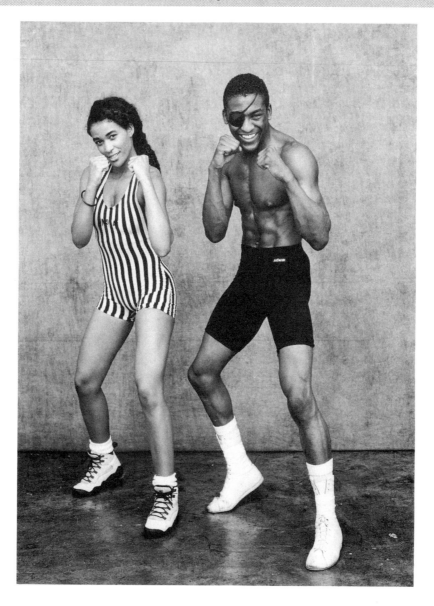

THE SUBJECT IS PARTNERS

Some of you may wonder about doing Aerobox with a partner.

In truth, I'm opposed to the notion.

This may seem a contradiction, given that I teach up to eight widely attended classes a week. So let me explain.

The spirit of boxing—from which Aerobox springs—is that of a solo endeavor. Similarly, those who take up Aerobox really are in competition with themselves.

My classes may have as many as forty men and women at once charging through their Aerobox exercises. But most of those folks got there on their own. And since the class was the only format in which Aerobox was initially offered, they had no Plan B to think about.

I will concede that doing Aerobox in a class offers one significant benefit. With dozens of men and women performing the same exercise, you have a handy visual reference of what each movement is supposed to look like. There is no shortage of technical cross-checking.

But the big picture is that you are really operating within yourself. When, say, you skip rope, you fall into a zone where nothing around you matters. The whirring of the rope, the light breeze its revolving action makes—all that wraps you within a peaceful cocoon. It's almost like you're floating. Everything else is far removed.

And I'm kind of partial to the serenity of the individual working hard in isolation.

But ...

I'm not you. And the partner you have in mind may be as steadfast as you in the desire for long-term fitness. That partner may be just what you need to keep to an Aerobox program.

If that's the case, I offer you and your partner this bonus: a few exercises built for two.

TOWEL DRILL

In this exercise for slipping punches, one of you will swing a towel in broad arcs—laterally or, simulating an uppercut, upward. The other individual slips under or to the side of the towel and follows the slip with a single punch and eventually two punches. The movements of both partners build in intensity ... and complexity. Then reverse roles so that both of you get a chance to dodge the towel.

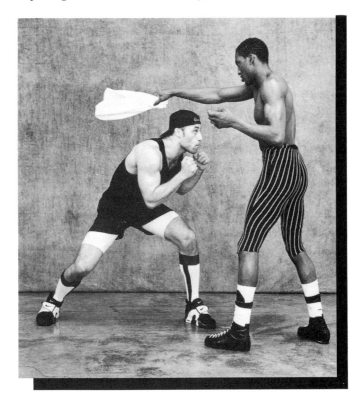

REMEMBER: if the towel is approaching from your left side, slip under to your left in a movement similar to the letter U.

NOTE: grip the towel by both ends so that you swing nothing but the blunt soft area. No edges, which can damage eyes.

COMPETITIVE ROPE

Real simple. Using a stopwatch, time an agreed-upon interval—like thirty or forty-five seconds—and count the number of revolutions each of you can do during that period. High number wins.

AIDED PUSH-UPS

At the end of a set, when their arms can barely support the barbell, weight-lifters have their partners help them get a last few repetitions. It's a profitable form of "cheating" in that the arm-weary lifter is still provoking the muscle, forcing it to do work that, while aided, draws benefits.

The same principle applies to aided push-ups. When you're struggling with your final repetitions, have your partner reach under your abs and help lift you through a few more teeth-clenching, blood-pumping push-ups.

THE TELEPHONE QUESTION

Q: What do I do if the phone rings while I'm in the middle of my Aerobox workout?

A: This is why God created answering machines. Let it ring.

FATHER KNOWS BEST

My father, Michael Olajidé, Sr., used to insist that I pay attention to my weak points when I was in the gym. "You can jab, you've got a good left hook," he'd say. "So work on your right hand."

That same principle applies to Aerobox.

Don't rush through the exercises that are more difficult for you. Work at them. And spend extra time if that's what it takes to get them right.

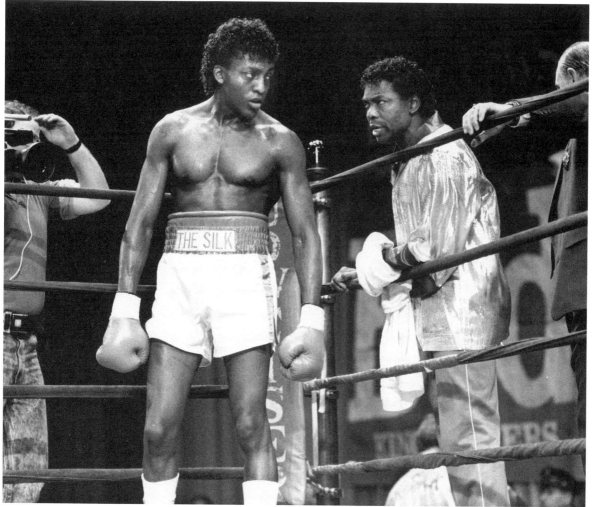

TOM CASINO

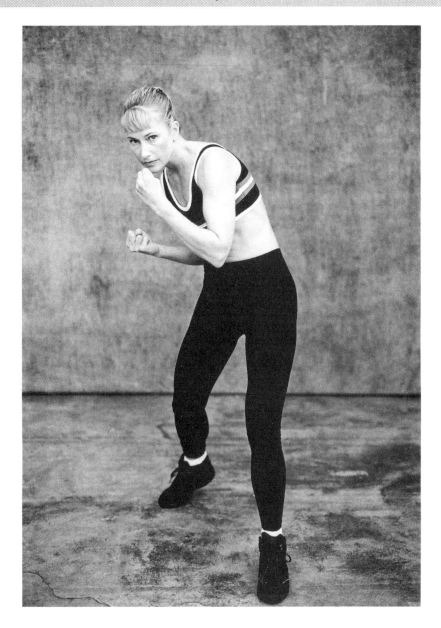

WOMEN IN AEROBOX, PART I

During my career, I fought a few guys who threw punches almost apologetically. Like they didn't want to hit you hard enough to provoke a real fight.

In Aerobox, women new to the program tend to have the same caution. Their timidity when they punch prevents them from getting full value from the exercise.

But that's because, by and large, they haven't the experience of punching other people. They've been conditioned to think of aggression of that sort as socially unacceptable.

For instance, when I tell the class to punch at an imagined opponent, guys throw their blows as if they see that foe in front of them. They punch as though they're trying to move something that's standing there.

Women don't. Not at first. They seem more concerned with tracking the contours of the punch ... with making the technical complexities manageable.

But most women slowly but surely lose their inhibitions about letting the punches go. Once they begin to vent their aggression, they come to like the feel of it. And that cliché of the weak female is transformed. Not only do their bodies become more defined through Aerobox, but their bearing changes too. They carry themselves more confidently—as though aware of and comfortable with the notion of newly found strength.

Where women have it over men in Aerobox is the experience of collective exercise. Over the last decade, women have taken aerobics classes and become accustomed to moving quickly and smartly through complicated physical maneuvers. What I find is that when men work from a stationary stance, they are adept at grasping combination punch sequences and then throwing those punches with a lot of steam behind them. But when those combination punches have more elaborate footwork mixed in, then women do better. Complex choreography is a snap for them.

Men are simply not used to the aerobics-class setting. Their preoccupation in health clubs tends to be with using weights to develop large anatomic contours. So many of them have big arms but haven't bothered to fine-tune the cardiovascular system. It's like having a Ferrari without an engine.

WOMEN IN AEROBOX, PART II

There are very specific concerns for women who take Aerobox—matters that, I think, are better addressed by an expert.

Dr. Laura MacIsaac, an obstetrician/gynecologist in a New York City hospital, has been doing Aerobox workouts for more than a year. Because of her familiarity with the program and her professional background, I asked her to discuss the issues important to women who were about to try Aerobox. Here are her comments.

Q: How and why can Aerobox help women?

A: After the age of thirty, women begin to lose bone density, a condition that can lead to problems when they grow older. Osteoporosis is the medical term for this weakening of the bones. Fifteen thousand women die from osteoporosis or its complications every year. For instance, femoral neck fractures are the twelfth leading cause of death for women in the United States, and those fractures occur when women suffer the trauma of falling down.

There are ways to slow the process and even increase bone density. The best way to increase bone density is in your younger years through weight-bearing and impact exercise and a good diet. That's why Aerobox is good for women in particular. Of course there are some women who have been told to stay away from strenuous programs like Aerobox and high-intensity step aerobics. But if you work those programs at your own pace, it shouldn't be a problem. And studies show that thirty minutes three times a week of weight-bearing exercise will increase the mineral content of bones in women aged forty to fifty.

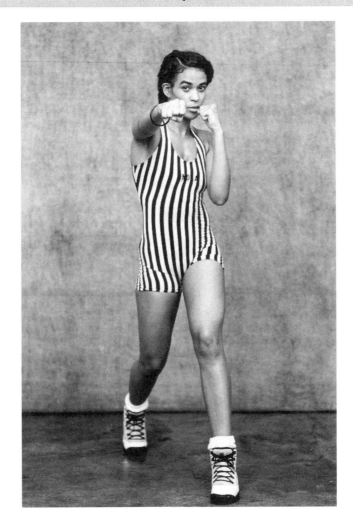

Our society imposes so many restrictions on women's ideas of self-image. One of the best ways to improve body image is to become stronger—not just look stronger but *feel* stronger. This entails a different kind of regimen rather than simply lifting weights or another vanity-oriented program. Through Aerobox, I have witnessed women improve their upper body awareness and as a result walk stronger, taller, with better posture, and new confidence and energy.

Q: What practical matters do women in particular need to be aware of when starting an Aerobox program?

A: Use a strong sports bra with extra support. It can be painful to jump rope without adequate breast support.

Avoid nylon bras and undergarments. They don't let the skin breathe, and sweating is therapeutic for the skin all over the body.

In weight-bearing exercises, every time there's impact or you jump, there's increased intra-abdominal pressure, which puts stress on a woman's bladder and urethra. This can cause transient incontinence—slight urination—and most typically occurs in women who have had children. It's why it's important for women to empty their bladder before doing any kind of vigorous exercise program, including Aerobox.

Q: What about pregnant women?

A: A woman may exercise when pregnant without fear of harm to the fetus as long as she does so at the same level she did before she became pregnant. The only exception is she doesn't want to become very overheated—more than 102 degrees—because temperatures greater than 102 in the first trimester have been associated with birth defects.

Q: So when should a woman stop her Aerobox program?

A: The logical answer is when the jarring from the jump rope becomes uncomfortable. This can be expected to occur at the last trimester—the final three months of pregnancy. But to be on the safe side, you'll want to consult your doctor regarding the specifics of your pregnancy.

Q: Are there special concerns for adolescents who take up Aerobox?

A: Adolescents engaged in a rigorous athletic program often have delayed menarche—onset of their menstrual cycle. But this has no adverse outcome, and the normal cycle will simply begin a little later. Adolescence is often a very difficult time for women because of their blossoming womanhood/sexuality. Exercise programs like Aerobox will actually greatly facilitate a young woman's growing into her body, and it has been shown that girls in competitive sports or exercise programs have an overall easier time with adolescence.

Q: Are there any problems a woman can anticipate when doing Aerobox during her period?

A: No. None at all. There should be no fear about doing Aerobox during a woman's period. In fact it has been shown that regular exercise is one of the best ways to improve symptoms of dysmenorrhea, the medical term for very painful periods.

SPOT TONING

While most folks undertake Aerobox to get fit, some of them have concerns about particular parts of their bodies. Their belly or butt may be too big, or they may want to lose the hanging flesh on the underside of the arms.

Whatever.

Aerobox does not offer spot-toning programs. But Aerobox over the long haul does generate retooled bodies.

To change fat, you have to change your metabolism. When you fatigue the body through exercise, it's like you're priming the body for metabolic change. Aerobox can, and does, activate the switch.

What's more, those who get the hang of Aerobox can eventually adapt the workouts to meet their specific body needs. Are you looking to take inches off your hips? Intensify your rope work and add on more punching while slipping punches—exercises that get

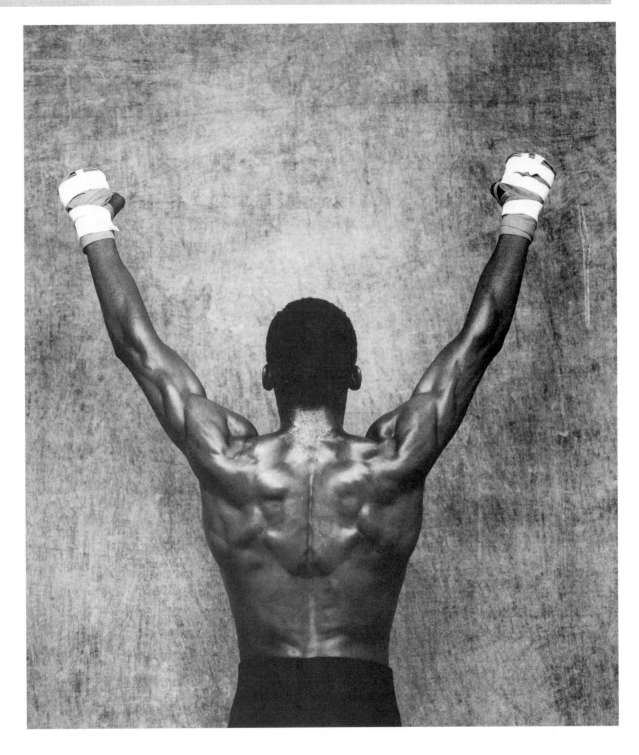

the glutes and thighs motivated. Want to firm the underside of your arms? Put in more time on the rope and rapid-fire punching sequences. Push-ups will help too. A firmer tummy? The rope, sit-ups, and torso twists in volume.

GOOD PAIN, BAD PAIN

Exercise is not pain-free.

When you work your body hard, you are often laboring on the rim of muscle fatigue.

That fatigue brings a certain sensation bordering on pain—a kind of sunburst of agony that, strangely enough, sometimes holds within it a pleasurable afterburn.

We all know that feeling of hard-won effort. It's pain that's worth pushing through.

But the twinge in the back, or knee, the slight seizure in your hamstring—these often are an SOS from a beleaguered body announcing that if you push the particular distressed area again, you are going to have problems.

The trick here is to learn what all the twinges and twitches of your particular body mean. You know the term—"listening to your body"? It's become a clichéd expression, but it's crucial, really, in any individual's long-term satisfaction with his exercise program.

The common cramp, or stitch, is the league-leading affliction in my classes. That pain in the side is often a result of fatigue from the workout combined with too much water intake, or of fatigue and the digestive tract's struggle with food eaten too close to workout time.

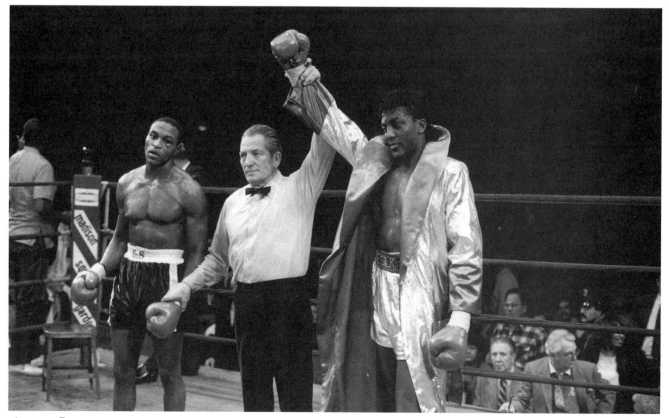

ANDREW BRUCKER

Nobody ever requires first aid for a stitch. It's the sort of fleeting pain that responds to reduced intensity, or possibly a temporary cessation, of exercise. Sometimes people just follow the gym teacher's ancient remedy for minor hurts: walk it off.

And in fact, that general principle—a go-slow caution—applies to any sudden sharp pain. Sometimes that shooting pain is no more than a quirky moment in the body's flow. Slowing down enables you to get a read on whether it's for real or not.

Don't be cavalier about your aches and pains. Be smart. Be sensitive.

THE IMPORTANCE OF THE CLENCHED FIST

Q: What happens if I punch with an open fist?

A: A loose hand tends to create a buggy-whip effect when you punch. In a worst-case scenario, that can cause you to hyperextend your elbow. Keep your fists closed.

ANOTHER INJURY CONCERN

You've been told that when slipping punches, you bend with the knees. But just as important is not to lock those knees when you raise up. Locking the knees wears on the joints and can lead to injuries.

BURNOUT

Burnout is a state of mental exhaustion.

As a fighter, I rubbed up against it in the unrelenting monotony of training ... and the nonstop focus on a career in a difficult business.

Aerobox, like any exercise program, comes with the same risks of growing stale.

The remedy is simple: variety.

Once you've grown accustomed to the beginner's and/or advanced workouts, you are not obliged to stick to the particulars ad infinitum.

Tinker with the workout, redesigning it from time to time to get the diversity that keeps you interested.

For those of you for whom Aerobox is your sole exercise, the answer may be to add another format—swimming, bicycling, jogging, even walking.

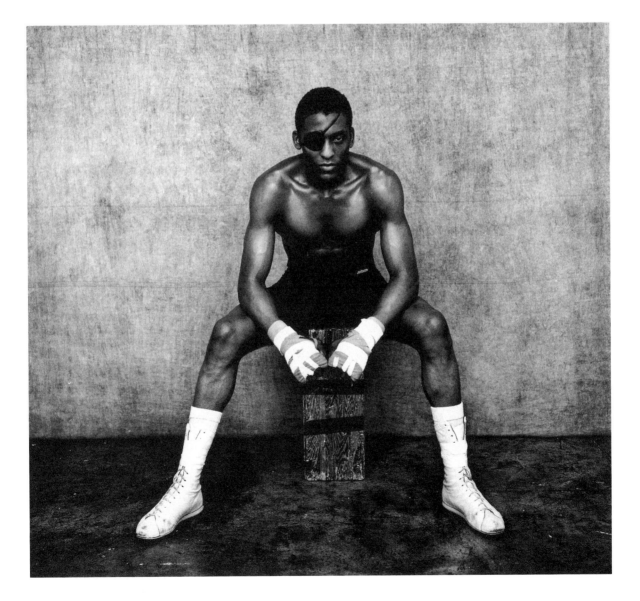

OLAJIDÉ ON OLAJIDÉ

I don't just talk my classes through the Aerobox workout. I punch, move, skip rope, and do all those push-ups and sit-ups as well.

It's how I earn my living now—and more. It's become my way of keeping up on a long-time interest in staying fit.

When I was a fighter, I prided myself on having more stamina than the next guy—a capability that I owed to the intense training I did.

These days, I do the Aerobox workout at least eight times a week. It's made my body more defined than when I was a fighter. That doesn't mean I'm in better shape now, just that at 163 pounds, three pounds more than the weight I fought at, I am somewhat more chiseled.

I may do the occasional set of pull-ups on a chinning bar, or leg presses and calf raises on weight machines, but mostly I rely on Aerobox to fulfill me.

You shouldn't think of me, though, as a natural-born physical specimen. When I was fifteen, I was skinny as a stick … so skinny, at ninety-six pounds, that when I played football in the public leagues in Vancouver, the competition routinely outweighed me by fifty to sixty pounds.

Nor was I especially athletic. I was cut from my school basketball team and was no blazing star as a running back and safety in those football leagues.

It was because of the weight inequity that I took up boxing. I figured that a sport in which I would be matched against fellows my size offered me the best chance to show what I could do.

I was lucky to have a father who had fought professionally in Nigeria and England, and had the patience and know-how to impart what he knew.

The rest had to do with hard work and that leap of faith that all of us take who dream of doing big things. Often it rubs up against the conventional thinking of those who think they know better.

I remember one day sitting with a friend at the kitchen table in my father's home. I was in my early teens and had begun to point toward a career in professional boxing. This friend wondered aloud about the possibility that I might not make it as a fighter— where would I be then? He suggested I ought to be prepared for the worst—and get whatever educational advantages would ensure a stable future.

My father was in earshot of this conversation, and wasn't happy with it. For he understood about that leap of faith dreamers take—and knew that my friend's notions were harmful to the psyche a fighter needed.

He told me afterward: "This is an attitude you are going to confront the rest of your life."

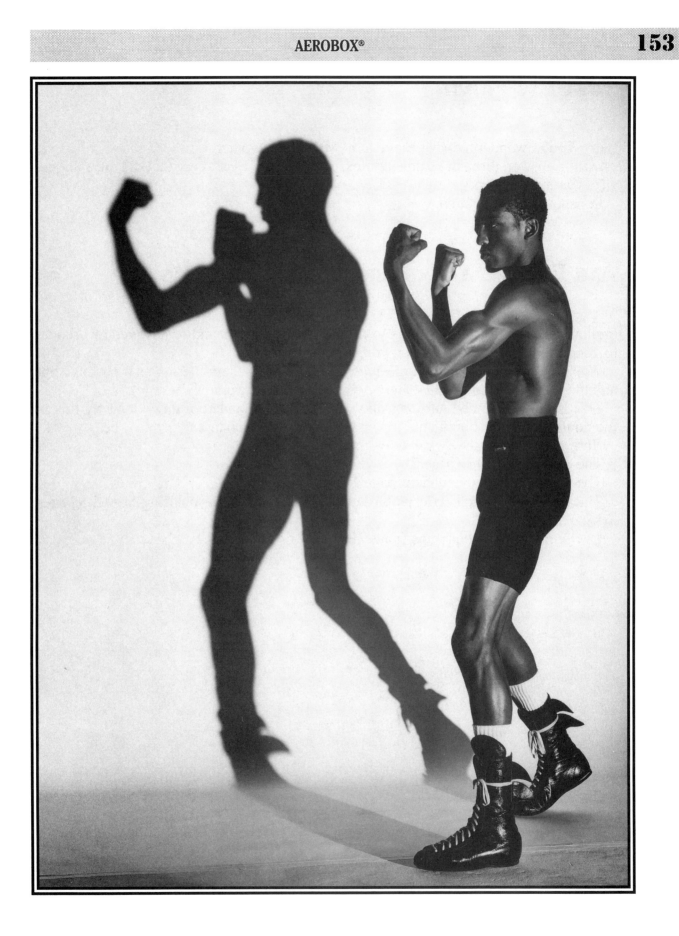

THAT EYE PATCH

Okay. You're wondering what the deal is with the eye patch.

Simple answer: through boxing injuries, compounded by surgery that did me a disservice, I've lost sight in the right eye.

Consequently, the patch.

AND FINALLY, YOUR AEROBOX TEST OF TESTS

Earlier, I suggested you might like to modify the beginner's and/or advanced workouts to keep them from going stale on you.

Well, for those out there who feel very ambitious . . . I am offering as a parting shot an elite gut-buster no-quiche-eaters-need-apply bonus workout.

This is ultra-advanced Aerobox, and you are warned ahead of time: don't try this in the confines of your home unless you are prepared to moan and groan a bit.

Here goes:

The Ankle Loosener (page 71)

The Opening Rope Sequence (page 109)

The Shoulder Stretch, Triceps Stretch, Calf Stretch, and Hamstring Stretch (pages 67–70)

12 Double-Bounce Push-ups (page 130).

STICK 'N' MOVE

POSITION: Boxer's stance.

MOVEMENT: On the balls of your feet, you bounce forward a step (count of one) and then bounce backward a step (count of two). Continue for 32 counts.

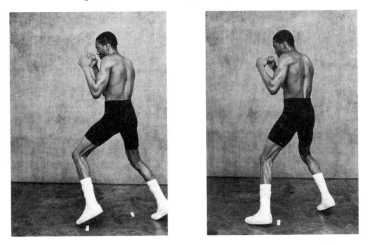

THE REST OF THE SEQUENCE: Repeat the movement. But as you come forward this time, throw a left jab. Continue to bounce forward and back, executing 32 jabs off the forward movement. Retract your jab before your back foot lands. Repeat the entire stick 'n' move sequence as a southpaw.

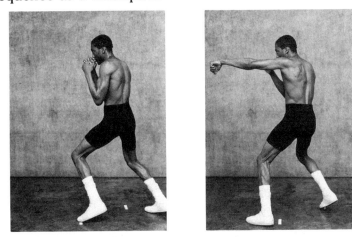

MUSCLES WORKED: Calves, biceps, pecs, and shoulder region.

12 Inverted Push-ups (page 96).

Quick Punch Series: From a boxer's stance, throw alternate lefts and rights, first 8 slow and then 16 fast. Those 24 punches constitute a set. Do 4 sets. Keep your abs tight. Your feet grip the ground firmly. Throw those 16 fast punches with intensity.

12 Thrust Push-ups (page 97).

Repeat the Quick Punch Series as a southpaw.

BOXER'S FINGERTIP PUSH-UPS

POSITION: Elevated on your toes, in the push-up position, hands under your shoulders. Your weight is supported by the fingertips and thumbs of both hands.

MOVEMENT: Lower yourself on those fingertips to within two to three inches of the floor, then rise up. Do 12.

MUSCLES WORKED: Deltoids, pecs, forearms, and the muscles of the hands. For boxers, these push-ups are calculated to diminish the risk of hand injuries.

The Twist-and-Punch Series (page 108). Note: every second day, do this portion of the elite workout as a southpaw.

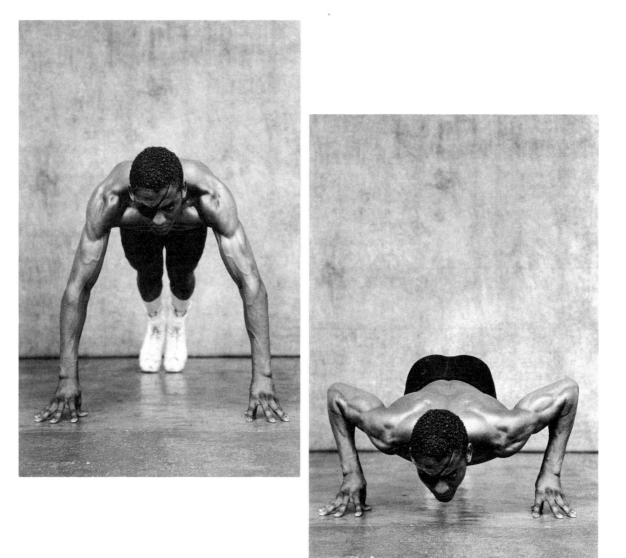

BODY SHOTS

POSITION: Boxer's stance.

MOVEMENT: Rather than directing your punches at the face of an imagined opponent, punch down toward an imagined body. Step and jab on one, noting that your step is an elongated one—almost like a fencer's thrusting movement. Count to yourself on two through eight. Do that eight-count maneuver 4 times.

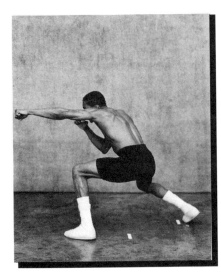 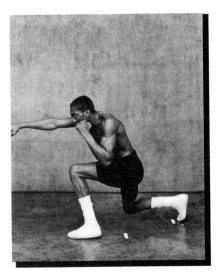

THE REST OF THE SEQUENCE: Step and throw a jab and right on one. Count two through eight. Do that 4 times. Then add another jab to the punching sequence and count two through eight for 4 sets. Add another right to the punching sequence and count two through eight for 4 sets. In the next phase, your sequence is jab-right, jab-right, jab-right, and count two through eight for 4 sets. Then jab-right, jab-right, jab-right, and count two through eight for 4 sets. Then elongate the sequence by adding a fourth jab, and count two through eight for 4 sets. Then add a final right hand, and count two through eight for 4 sets. Repeat the whole sequence as a southpaw.

MUSCLES WORKED: Glutes, quads, and the shoulder region.

Rope Sequence No. 2: Side-to-side figure eights for 16 counts (page 80), 32 basic jumps (page 81), 32 boxer's skips with rope (page 111), 16 basic jumps, 32 downhills (page 82), 16 basic jumps. Now drop the rope.

64 V-slips from a right-handed stance, executed quickly (page 78).

Rope Sequence No. 3: 32 basic jumps; 32 Aerobox run (page 86); the 911 (page 116)—for fifteen seconds every jump is at an accelerated pace, then you do fifteen seconds of basic jumps, fifteen seconds of 911, and the final fifteen seconds of basic jumps; 16 boxer's skips. Drop the rope.

64 V-slips from a southpaw stance, executed quickly.

Rope Sequence No. 4: 32 basic jumps; ankle touches (page 118); 16 basic jumps.

KNEE LIFTS

POSITION: Squared-off stance, holding the rope by the handles.

MOVEMENT: As you jump, bring your knee up to your chest, using your abs to help you lift it. This movement closely resembles what chorus lines do in Las Vegas and on the stage of Radio City Music Hall. Begin with the right leg, and alternate right and left for 32 knee lifts. Then double up the lifts: right-right and left-left for a total of 16.

MUSCLES WORKED: Glutes, abs, and calves.

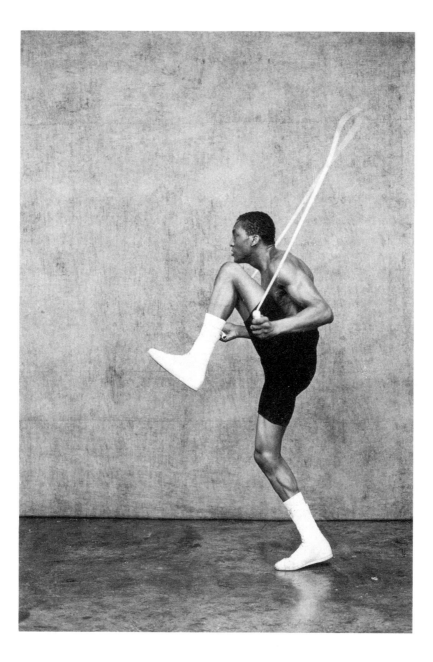

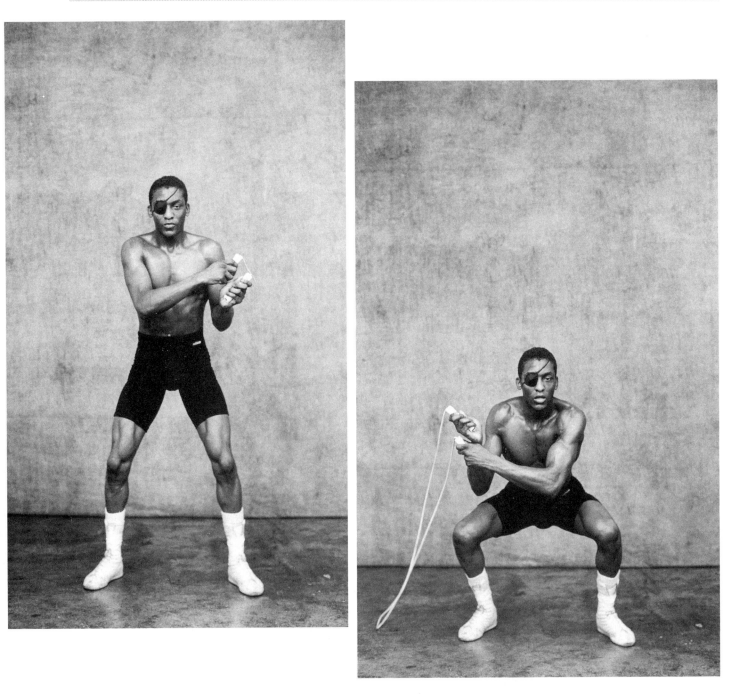

Rope Sequence No. 5: 16 basic jumps; slow side-to-side figure eights with a half squat every time you bring the rope to the right side (16 half squats in all); slow side-to-side figure eights with a half squat every time you bring the rope to either side (64 half squats in all); 16 basic jumps; 64 advanced speed skating jumps (page 115); 16 double-bounce speed-skating jumps; 16 basic jumps; 64 double jumps from the advanced workout (page 117); 16 basic jumps; 16 boxer's skips. Put the rope down.

64 Quick Feet (page 107) and then 64 Quick Feet moving laterally instead of forward and back. Repeat both segments as a southpaw.

RESISTANCE PUSH-UPS

POSITION: Lie on your stomach, with your hands beneath your chest. Your fingers are flared, the sides of the thumbs touching. The toes point into the ground as you elevate your body.

MOVEMENT: What you are doing are thumbs-touch push-ups (page 95) in a kind of slow motion. Lower yourself and, without touching the ground, hold your body two to three inches aloft for sixteen seconds. Then rise up and at the apex of the movement hold for eight seconds. Do that up-and-down sequence 3 times.

THE REST OF THE SEQUENCE: What you are now doing are inverted push-ups (fingers facing in, elbows flaring out—page 96) in a kind of slow motion. Perform them to the specifications just used for the resistance thumbs-touch push-ups. Your hands will be set wide. When both resistance push-ups are done, take a thirty-second break as a lead-in to . . .

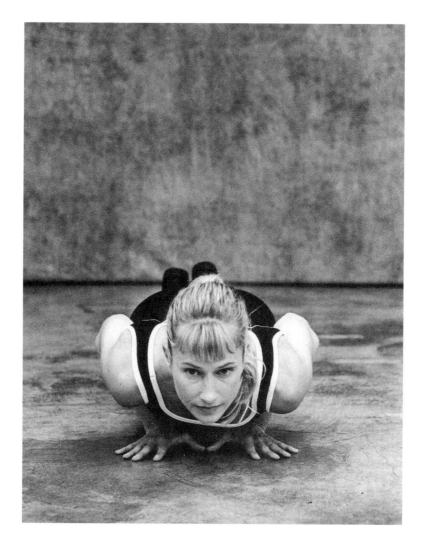

BOXER'S ONE-ARM PUSH-UPS

POSITION: You are elevated sideways to the ground, your weight supported by your right arm. The right hand is inverted, facing to the left. The left hand is either on your hip or (as an option to make the push-up somewhat easier) with fingertips cupped against the ground.

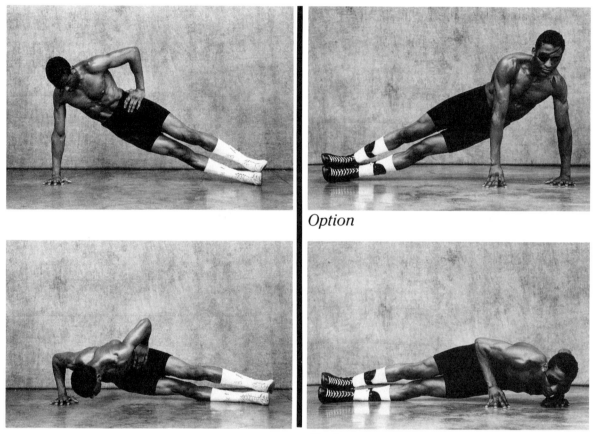

Option

Option

MOVEMENT: Lower your upper body down, but don't touch the ground. Only your hand(s) and feet should be touching the ground. Keep your right shoulder pointing to the ceiling. Don't square up your body. Lower sideways until you're two inches from the ground, then rise up. Do 8 one-arm push-ups on each arm.

MUSCLES WORKED: Rear and front deltoids, pecs and triceps.

64 Neck Nods (page 120); 64 Neck Nods (but laterally rather than up and down); Alternating-Leg Ab Crunches (page 93); Swivel Leg Extensions (pages 122–123); Aerobox Crunch 'n' Punch (pages 90–91); Lateral V-sits (double the specifications—page 125).

KNEE HUGS

POSITION: You're on your back, left leg extended, right leg bent at the knee and, initially, your right foot flat to the ground.

MOVEMENT: Clasp your right leg just below the knee and pull your knee off the ground toward your head, which is raised off the ground. Hold for twelve seconds. Repeat with the other leg.

MUSCLES WORKED: Lower back and glutes.

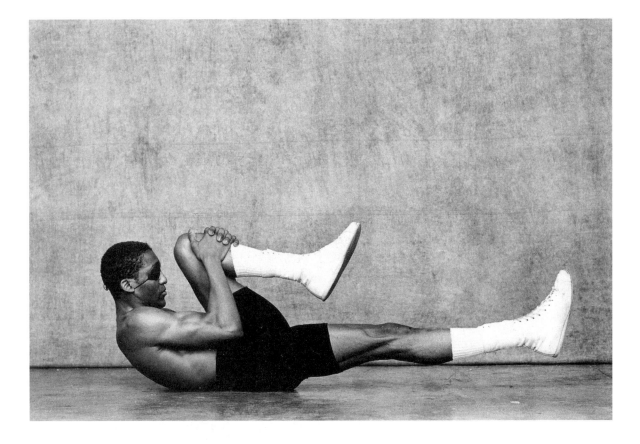

LAID-BACK FIGURE-FOUR

POSITION: You're on your back. The right leg is bent at the knee and your right foot is flat to the ground. The left foot is placed above the right knee and extends just beyond it.

MOVEMENT: Place your left hand on your left knee and push down from the inside of the knee. Hold that stretch for twelve seconds. Release for six seconds and then push the knee down again for twelve seconds. Change legs and repeat.

MUSCLES WORKED: Hip flexors.

Do the Ab Stretch (page 94), the Lat Stretch, the Shoulder Stretch, the Calf Stretch, the Hamstring Stretch, and the Lower Back Stretch (pages 98–102).

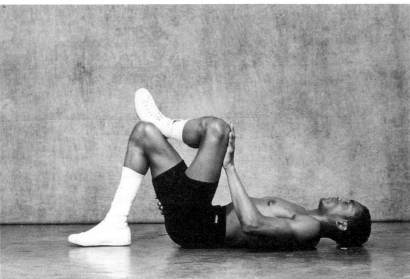

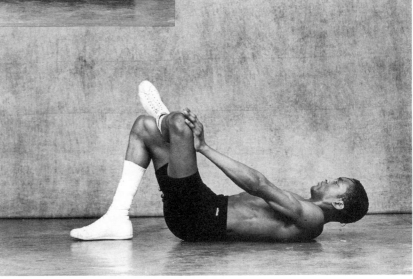

AEROBOX LEVITATION STRETCH

POSITION: You're seated, with your knees flared and the bottoms of your feet touching. Your hands clasp the top portion of your feet.

MOVEMENT: Take a deep breath, inhaling through your nose, and straighten your back, looking up to the ceiling. Hold for twelve seconds, stretching your trapezius.

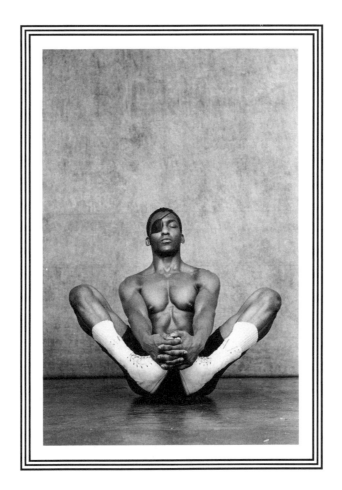

THE REST OF THE SEQUENCE: Exhale and pull with your hands so that your head lowers toward your feet. Hold for twelve seconds, stretching your upper back. Now, as you inhale through the nose, rise up, straightening your back so that your feet come off the ground. The effect is as though you're levitating. Actually, your feet are off the ground and you're balanced on your buttocks. Hold that for thirty-two seconds. It's more a calming movement than a stretch. Inhale on one, exhale on two through eight.

This marks the end of the elite Aerobox workout.

GLOSSARY

Aerobox—(pronounced air-ROW-box) The ultimate noncontact boxing workout, created by Michael Olajidé, Jr., a former professional world-ranked fighter.

Combination—A sequence of several punches, executed with both hands.

Crossing the Rope—An advanced skip-rope technique in which an individual flicks his wrists at each other and creates a loop big enough to jump through.

Crunches—A sit-up done in a tight, controlled arc of about nine inches.

Feint—A boxing maneuver employing the head or shoulders, hands or feet, calculated to fake the opponent out of position while creating an opening for a punch.

Figure Eights—A pattern created while standing in place and turning the rope by rolling both wrists. Done correctly, the rope makes an X in front and loops at the side—the portrait of that eight.

Hook—A power punch thrown in a lateral arc with either hand.

Jab—The punch used to probe the opponent's defense, creating the openings for heavier punches.

Pyramid Position—The placement of hands—each to the side of the jaw—when taking up the boxer's stance.

Set Position—The position a fighter takes—both hands up and one foot in advance of the other—before he strikes.

Slipping—The art of eluding punches.

The Old One-Two—A punching combination of the jab followed by a straight right hand thrown with bad intentions.

Torque—The force added to a punch by twisting the hips and shoulders into it.

Uppercut—A power punch thrown in an upward arc with either hand.

INDEX

Page numbers of illustrations are set in italics.

A

Abbreviated 911, 116, *116*
Abdominals (abs), exercises for, *40. See also* Obliques
  abbreviated 911, 116, *116*
  advanced rapid-rope series, 114
  Aerobox crunch 'n' punch, 90-92, *90-91*
  Aerobox run, 86-87, *86*
  alternating-leg ab crunches, 93, *93*
  crunches, 89, *89*
  elevated-leg ab crunches, 92, *92*
  knee-lifts, 158, *158*
  lateral slip, 24
  lower back stretch, 102, *102*
  push-up, 39, 42
  right-hand power punch, 14, 15, 74, *74*
  sit-ups, 39, 42
  stretch, 94, *94*
  twisting ab crunches, 121, *121*
  V-sits, 124, *124*
Ab stretch, 94, *94*
Advanced multi-punch series
  no. 1, 111
  no. 2, 112, *112*
Advanced rapid-rope series, 114
Advanced workout, 105-6
  advanced rapid-rope series, 114-18
  body toning exercises, 120-31
  cool down, 119
  opening rope sequence, 109-11
  punch series, 111-14
  stretches, 132-36
  warm-up, 106-8
Aerobox, xi, 165. *See also* Advanced Workout; Beginners
    Workout; Elite Workout
  benefits, xi, 3, 42, 80
  diversity of workout, 42
  exercise blocks in, 4
  frequency of workouts, 3, 59
  as full-body workout, 3, 42
  length of workout session, 4
  objectives, 39
  succession of movements, 26
  as supplementary workout, 59
  what to expect, 51-52

Aerobox crunch 'n' punch, 90-92, *90, 91*
Aerobox levitation stretch, 164, *164*
Aerobox run, 86-87, *86*
Agility, 80
  ankle cross jumps, 85, *85*
Aided push-ups, 142
Ali lean, 25, *25,* 107
Ali, Muhammad, xi
  fights of, 28
  style, 107
Ali, Nelson, 49-50
Ali shuffle, xii, 34, *34*
Alternating-leg ab crunches, 93, *93*
Ambidexterity, 36
Ankle, exercises for
  boxer's skip (with rope), 111
  loosener, 71, *71*
  toe raises, 62
Ankle cross jumps, 85, *85*
Ankle touches, 118, *118*
Arms, exercises for. *See also* specific muscles
  definition and toning, 10
  skipping rope, 36

B

Back (lower) exercises
  knee hug, 162, *162*
  stretch, 102, *102*
Back (upper) exercises
  hook, 16, 75, *75*
  lateral slip and counters, 78
  right-hand power punch, 14, 74, *74*
  shoulder stretch, 67, *67*
  sitting series stretch, 132-36, *132-36*
  V-slips and counters, 78
Balance, 22
Barkley, Iran (The Blade), 19
Beginner's workout, 61-62
  advanced exercises to supplement, 105
  cool-down (stretching), 87, 98-104
  jump rope, 80-87
  punching, 72-77
  slips and counters, 78-79
  toning, 87-98
  warm-up exercises, 62-71
Biceps, exercises for, *40*
  double-bounce push-ups, 130, *130*

(Biceps, exercises for, continued.)
double jumps and more rapid rope, 117
hook, 16, 75, *75*
jab, 9, 72-73, *73*
push-up, 39, 42
stick 'n' move, 155, *155*
uppercut, 17, 76, *77*
V-slips and counters, 78
Body shots, 157, *157*
Boxer's fingertip push-ups, 156, *156*
Boxer's one-arm push-ups, 161, *161*
Boxer's skip
without rope, 106
with rope, 111
Boxing matches. *See also* specific fighters
fatigue during, 54
first round, 53
Breathing
exercise, 164
heavy, 53-54
Bruno, Frank, 28
Burnout, 151
Buttocks exercise
downhill jumps, 82

C

Calf stretch, 69, *69*
Calves, exercises for
abbreviated 911, 116, *116*
advanced rapid-rope series, 114
Ali lean, 25, *25*, 107
ankle cross jumps, 85, *85*
ankle touches, 118, *118*
boxer's skip (without rope), 106
boxer's skip (with rope), 111
double jumps and more rapid rope, 117
downhill jumps, 82
feint and fire, 119
footwork, 21
jumping jacks, 84, *84*
knee-lifts, 158, *158*
one-footed hops, 81-82, *81*
opening rope sequence, advanced, 109, *109*
quick feet, 107
side-to-side figure eights, 80-81
sitting series stretch, 132-36, *132-36*
skipping rope, 29, 36
stick 'n' move, 155, *155*
stretch, 69, *69*, 100, *100*
toe raises, 62
Cardiovascular exercises, xi
accelerated pulse/heavy breathing, 53-54, 79
Aerobox run, 86-87, *86*
side-to-side figure eights, 80-81
skipping rope, 29, 36, 80
Chávez, Julio César, 16
Clothing for workout, *57,* 57-58
women, 146
Coetzer, Pierre, 10
Combination punching, 10, 79, 111-14, 165

Concentration, 26
Cool-down
beginners, 87-88, 98-104
side-steps, 87
twist-and punch, 88, *88*
Coordination, 18, 23, 80
ankle cross jumps, 85, *85*
Counterpunching, 26, 53, 78-79
Cramp or stitch, 149-50
Crossing the rope, 110, 165
Crunches, 89, *89,* 165. *See also* Abdominals; Obliques; Sit-ups

D

D'Amato, Cus, 8
Deltoids (front and rear), exercises for, *40, 41*
boxer's fingertip push-ups, 156, *156*
boxer's one-arm push-ups, 161, *161*
inverted push-ups, *39,* 96, *96*
jab, 9, 10, 72-73, *73*
lateral slip and counters, 78
push-up, 39, 42
shoulder stretch, 67, *67,* 99, *99*
shovel push-ups, 128, *128-29*
side-to-side figure eights, 80-81
sitting series stretch, 132-36, *132-36*
skipping rope, 29
thrust push-ups, 97, *97*
thumbs-touch push-ups, 95, *95*
tricep sits, 131, *131*
V-slips and counters, 78
DeWitt, Doug, xii
Double-bounce push-ups, 130, *130*
Double jumps, 36, *36*
Double jumps and more rapid rope, 117
Douglas, James (Buster), 18, 28
self-destructiveness, 55-56
Downhill jumps, 82
Duran, Roberto
and jab, 12
and jump rope, 37
and mind games/defeat of, 56

E

Eating before workout, 58, 149
Elevated-leg ab crunches, 92, *92*
Elite workout
body toning, 160-61
opening rope sequence, 154
punch series, 155, 156-57
push-ups, 154, 155, 156, 160-61
rope sequences, 157-60
stretching, 162-64
warm-up, 154
Equipment needed for workout, xii, 4, 57-59
Exercise blocks, 4

F

Face muscles, exercise
  neck nods, 120, *120*
Fat, body
  aerobic conditioning for loss, 80
  Aerobox and metabolism, 147
  spot toning, 147-48
Fatigue
  during boxing matches, 54
  during workout, 54
Fear, and punching, 8
Feet
  boxer's skip (with rope), 111
  side-to-side figure eights, 80-81
  skipping rope, 29
  toe raises, 62
Feint, 165
Feint and fire, 119
Figure Eights, 165
Figure four stretch, 103, *103*
Fist
  importance of clenched, 150
  for jab, 10
  making a, 8
"Flip Fantasia" (Us3), 59
Footwear recommended, 58
Footwork, 21-28, *21, 22. See also* Jump rope; specific moves
Forearms, exercises for, *40*
  boxer's fingertip push-ups, 156, *156*
  definition and toning, 10
  double jumps and more rapid rope, 117
  opening rope sequence, advanced, 109, *109*
  side-to-side figure eights, 80-81
  skipping rope, 29, 36
Foreman, George
  and jab, 10, 12
  and power punches, 19
Foster, Bob, 19
Frazier, Joe
  footwork, 28
  and hook, 16

G

Gastrocnemius muscle, exercises for, *41*
  advanced rapid-rope series, 114
  calf stretch, 69, *69*
Gluteus maximus and lateral (glutes), exercises for, *41*
  abbreviated 911, 116, *116*
  Aerobox run, 86-87, *86*
  body shots, 157, *157*
  combination punching, 79
  downhill jumps, 82
  footwork, 21, 23
  jumping jacks, 84, *84*
  knee hug, 162, *162*
  knee-lifts, 158, *158*
  lateral V-sits, 125, *125*

  opening rope sequence, advanced, 109, *109*
  quick feet, 107
  skipping rope, 34, 36
  slip twist-and-punch, 65-67, *65, 66*
  V-slips and counters, 78
  yoga stretch, 104, *104*
Green, James (Hard Rock), 56
Groin area
  figure four stretch, 103, *103*

H

Hamstring exercises, *41*
  advanced rapid-rope series, 114
  Aerobox run, 86-87, *86*
  sitting series stretch, 132-36, *132-36*
  speed skating, 115, *115*
  stretches, 70, *70,* 101, *101*
Hamstring stretch, 70, *70,* 101, *101*
Hands (and metacarpals), exercises for
  boxer's fingertip push-ups, 156, *156*
  fingertip push-up, 39
Head movements, 25, 28
Hearns, Thomas, xi, *12, 13*
  and jab, 12
  and power punches, 19
Heiden, Eric, 115
Hip flexors, exercises for
  laid-back figure-four, 163, *163*
  sitting series stretch, 132-36, *132-36*
Hips, exercises for
  downhill jumps, 82
  sitting series stretch, 132-36, *132-36*
Holmes, Larry, 10
Holyfield, Evander, 18, 56
  on mind/attitude, 55
  on training, 43
Hook, *16,* 16-17, 165
  left, 75, *75*

I

Injury, concerns about, 149-50
  hand, 156
Inverted push-ups, 96, *96*
Inverted triceps push-ups, 127, *127*
Irish jig, 35, *35*

J

Jab, *9,* 9-12, 165
  beginner's workout, 72-73, *73*
  footwork for, 22, *22,* 23, *23*
  "hang," 73
  "lazy," 73

Johnson, John, 56
Jumping jacks, 84, *84*
Jump rope, 29-37
   abbreviated 911, 116, *116*
   accelerated pulse/shortness of breath during, 53-54
   advanced rapid-rope series, 114
   Aerobox run, 86-87, *86*
   Ali shuffle, 34, *34*
   ambidexterity, 36
   ankle cross jumps, 85, *85*
   ankle touches, 118, *118*
   boxer's skip, 111
   competitive rope, 142
   crossing the rope, 33, *33,* 110, 165
   double jump, 36, *36*
   double jumps and more rapid rope, 117
   downhill jumps, 82
   elite workout, 154, 157-60
   half-squats with figure eight, 159, *159*
   Irish jig, 35, *35*
   jumping jacks, 84, *84*
   knee-lifts, 158, *158*
   length, determining, *30,* 30-31
   with mirror, 4-5
   Olajidé on, 36-37
   one-footed hops, 81-82, *81*
   opening sequence, advanced, 109, *109*
   pivot jumps, 83, *83*
   sideways jumps/side-to-side figure eights, 34, *34,* 80-81
   speed skating, 115, *115*
   technique, 32, *32*
   type to use, 29, 80
   warming up, 31, *31*
   warnings, 80
   and workout order, 37

K

Kalambay, Sumbu, 50
Kingsway Boxing Gym, 11
Knee hugs, 162, *162*
Knee lifts, 158, *158*
Knees
   bending for slipping punches, 26
   injury, 150

L

Laid-back figure-four, 163, *163*
Lateral slip, 24, *24*
   and counters, 78
Latissimus dorsi muscle (lats), exercises for, 12, *41*
   inverted push-ups, *39,* 96, *96*
   push-up, 39, 42
   right-hand power punch, 14, 74, *74*
   shoulder stretch, 99, *99*
   shovel push-ups, 128, *128-29*
   stretch, 98, *98*

   thrust push-ups, 97, *97*
   thumbs-touch push-ups, 95, *95*
   tricep stretch, *43,* 68, *68*
   uppercut, 17, 76, *77*
   V-slips and counters, 78
Lat stretch, 98, *98*
Left-handers (southpaws)
   for jab, 10
   stance, 8, *64,* 65, *65*
   and straight right hand punch, 14
Left hook. *See* Hook
Leonard, Sugar Ray, 56
Legs. *See also* specific muscles
   footwork, 21
Liston, Sonny
   and jab, 12
   and power punches, 19
Lord G., 58
"Love and Happiness" (Us3), 59
Lower back stretch, 102

M

MacIsaac, Laura, 145-47
McSwain, Stacy, 50
Men and Aerobox, xii, 145
Metacarpals. *See* Hands
Mind (and attitude) in boxing, 49-50, 55-56
Mirror, use of, 4, 11, 26
Movement. *See also* Slipping punches
   principles of, 22
   stick 'n' move, 155, *155*
Muscle groups, *40-41. See also* specific muscles
   midsection, 79, 83
   upper body, 79
Muscle soreness, 52, 149-50
Music, adding to workout, xii, 58-59

N

Neck nods, 120, *120*
New York Jets, xii

O

Obliques, exercises for, *40*
   Aerobox crunch 'n' punch, 90-92, *90-91*
   Ali lean, 25, *25,* 107
   alternating-leg ab crunches, 93, *93*
   hook, 16, 75, *75*
   lateral slip, 24
   lateral slip and counters, 78
   lateral V-sits, 125, *125*
   lower back stretch, 102, *102*
   sitting series stretch, 132-36, *132-36*

sit-ups, 39, 42
slip twist-and-punch, 65-67, *65, 66*
swivel leg extensions, 122, *122-23*
torso twists, 63-64, *63, 64*
twist-and-punch series, 108
twisting ab crunches, 121, *121*
twisting oblique stretch, 126, *126*
uppercut, 17, 76, *77*
V-slips and counters, 78
Olajidé, Michael
  as amateur boxer, 49
  boyhood, 152
  on footwork, *27,* 27-28
  decision to enter boxing, 152
  early training in Vancouver, 3-4, 19
  eye patch, xi, 154
  on jab, 11-12
  on jump rope, 37
  on mind and attitude, 50, 55-56
  on movement, 22
  nickname, 27
  physical condition/physique today, 152
  on power punches, 19
  professional career/fights, xi, 12, *12, 13,* 50, 53-54
  stamina, 152
  on training work ethic, 45, 50
Olajidé, Sr., Michael (father), 3, 11, 143, *143,* 152
Olajidé special combination series, 113-14, *113*
"Old one-two," 12, 14, 165
One-footed hops, 81-82, *81*
Orbital 2 album, 59

P

Pace, setting a, xii, 11
Pain, 149-50
Parker, Curtis, 53-54
Partners, 140-41
  aided push-ups, 142
  competitive rope, 142
  towel drill, 141-42, *141-42*
Pectorals, exercises for, *40*
  advanced rapid-rope series, 114
  boxer's fingertip push-ups, 156, *156*
  boxer's one-arm push-ups, 161, *161*
  crossing the rope, 110
  double-bounce push-ups, 130, *130*
  double jumps and more rapid rope, 117
  fingertip push-up, 39
  inverted push-ups, *39,* 96, *96*
  inverted triceps push-ups, 127, *127*
  jab, 9, 10, 72-73, *73*
  lateral slip and counters, 78
  push-up, 39, 42
  right-hand power punch, 14, 74, *74*
  shovel push-ups, 128, *128-29*
  side-to-side figure eights, 80-81
  skipping rope, 29, 36
  stick 'n' move, 155, *155*
  thrust push-ups, 97, *97*
  thumbs-touch push-ups, 95, *95*

twist-and-punch series, 108
  V-slips and counters, 78
Pep, Willie, 21-22
Pivot jumps, 83, *83*
Pull-ups for V body shape, 19
Punching, 7-19. *See also* specific fighters; specific punches
  advanced workout, 108, 111-14
  and back, 19
  beginner's workout, 72-77
  combinations, 10
  elite workout, 155, 156-57
  and fatigue, 13-14
  making a fist, 8
  power punches, 13-14, 19
  pull-ups recommended for, 19
  stance, *3, 7,* 7-8
  telegraphing, 72
  and tension, 8
  torque, need for, 15, 165
Push-ups, 39, *39,* 42
  aided, 142
  boxer's fingertip, 156, *156*
  boxer's one-arm, 161, *161*
  double-bounce, 130, *130*
  fingertip, 39, 42
  inverted, *39,* 96, *96*
  inverted triceps, 127, *127*
  resistance, 160, *160*
  shovel, 128, *128-29*
  standard military, 42
  thrust, 97, *97*
  thumbs-touch, 95, *95*
  tricep sits, 131, *131*
Pyramid position, *3, 7,* 8, 165

Q

Quadriceps (quads), exercises for, *40*
  body shots, 157, *157*
  combination punching, 79
  downhill jumps, 82
  feint and fire, 119
  footwork, 21, 23
  opening rope sequence, advanced, 109, *109*
  skipping rope, 36
  slip twist-and-punch, 65-67, *65, 66*
  speed skating, 115, *115*
  V-slips and counters, 78
Quick feet, 107

R

Resistance push-ups, 160, *160*
"Riding a punch," 25
Right-hand power punch, 14-15, *14, 15,* 74, *74*
Robinson, Sugar Ray, xi
  footwork, 28
  and jump rope, 37

Rotor cuffs exercise
    push-up, 39, 42

S

Serratus muscle, *40*
Set position, 22, 165
Setting (area needed) for workout, 58-59
Shadow boxing, 10
Shoulder blades exercise
    shoulder stretches, 67, *67,* 99, *99*
Shoulders, exercises for
    body shots, 157, *157*
    crossing the rope, 110
    double-bounce push-ups, 130, *130*
    double jumps and more rapid rope, 117
    shovel push-ups, 128, *128-29*
    sitting series stretch, 132-36, *132-36*
    skipping rope, 36
    slip twist-and-punch, 65-67, *65, 66*
    stick 'n' move, 155, *155*
    stretch, 67, *67,* 99, *99*
    torso twists, 63-64, *63, 64*
    twist-and-punch series, 108
Shoulder shrugs, 62
Shoulder stretches, 67, *67,* 99, *99*
Shovel push-ups, 128, *128-29*
Side steps, 87
Side-to-side figure eights, 80-81
Sitting series stretch, 132-36, *132-36*
Sit-ups (and crunches), 39, 42
    Aerobox crunch 'n' punch, 90-92, *90-91*
    alternating-leg ab crunches, 93, *93*
    crunches, 89, *89*
    elevated-leg ab crunches, 92, *92*
    form tip, 42
    lateral V-sits, 125, *125*
    swivel leg extensions, 122, *122-23*
    twisting ab crunches, 121, *121*
    V-sits, 124, *124*
Skipping rope. *See* Jump rope
Slipping punches, 165
    Ali lean, 25, *25,* 107
    feint and fire, 119
    knees, bending at, 26
    lateral slip, 24, *24,* 78
    slip twist-and-punch, 65-67, *65, 66*
    towel drill, 141-42, *141-42*
    twist-and-punch series, 108
    V-slip, 23, *23,* 78
Slip twist-and-punch, 65-67, *65, 66*
Soleus, exercises for, *41*
    ankle touches, 118, *118*
    boxer's skip (with rope), 111
    calf stretch, 69, *69*
    jumping jacks, 84, *84*
    one-footed hops, 81-82, *81*
    quick feet, 107
    side-to-side figure eights, 80-81
    skipping rope, 29
    toe raises, 62

Sparring, 4
Speed skating, 115, *115*
Spinks, Michael, 28
Stamina, 80
Stance, *3, 7,* 7-8, 22, *22, 61*
    jab, 10
    right-hand power punch, 14-15
    southpaw (left-hand), 8, *64,* 65, *65*
Stick 'n' move, 155, *155*
Straight right hand punch. *See* Right-hand power punch
Stretching (and limbering)
    ab stretch, 94, *94*
    Aerobox levitation stretch, 164
    ankle loosener, 71, *71*
    calf stretches, 69, *69,* 100, *100*
    figure four stretch, 103
    hamstring stretches, 70, *70,* 101, *101*
    and injury, 44
    knee hug, 162, *162*
    laid-back figure-four, 163, *163*
    lat stretch, 98, *98*
    lower back stretch, 102, *102*
    shoulder stretches, 67, *67,* 99, *99*
    sitting series, 132-36, *132-36*
    triceps stretch, *43,* 68, *68*
    twisting oblique stretch, 126, *126*
    warm-down, 44
    warm-up, 43-44
    yoga stretch, 104
Swivel leg extensions, 122, *122-23*

T

Telegraphing a punch, 72
Thighs, exercises for
    lateral V-sits, 125, *125*
    side-to-side figure eights, 80-81
    skipping rope, 29, 34
Thighs, inner, exercises for
    figure four stretch, 103, *103*
    sitting series stretch, 132-36, *132-36*
Thrust push-ups, 97, *97*
Thumbs-touch push-ups, 95, *95*
Tips
    difficult exercises, 143
    sit-ups form, 42
    telephone interruption, 142
Toe raises, 62
Toning, 39, 42, 80
    advanced workout, 120-31
    beginners workout, 87-98
    elite workout, 160-61
    push-ups, 39
    spot, 147-48
Torque, 13, 165
    and hook, 17
    right-hand power punch, 15, 74, *74*
Torso twists, 63-64, *63, 64*
Towel drill, 141-42, *141-42*
Trapezius (traps), exercises for, *41*
    Aerobox levitation stretch, 164
    jab, 9, 10, 72-73, *73*

lateral slip and counters, 78
right-hand power punch, 14, 74, *74*
shoulder shrugs, 62
side-to-side figure eights, 80-81
skipping rope, 29
uppercut, 17, 76, *77*
V-slips and counters, 78
yoga stretch, 104, *104*
Triceps, exercises for, *41*
  boxer's one-arm push-ups, 161, *161*
  double-bounce push-ups, 130, *130*
  inverted push-ups, *39*, 96, *96*
  inverted triceps push-ups, 127, *127*
  jab, 9, 10, 72-73, *73*
  lat stretch, 98, *98*
  push-up, 39, 42
  right-hand power punch, 14, 74, *74*
  shoulder stretch, 67, *67*
  shovel push-ups, 128, *128-29*
  sits, 131, *131*
  sitting series stretch, 132-36, *132-36*
  stretch, *43*, 68, *68*
  thrust push-ups, 97, *97*
  thumbs-touch push-ups, 95, *95*
  twist-and-punch series, 108
  V-slips and counters, 78
Triceps sits, 131, *131*
Triceps stretch, *43*, 68, *68*
"Tukka Yoots Riddim" (Us3), 59
Twist-and-punch, 88, *88*
  series, 108
Twisting ab crunches, 121, *121*
Twisting oblique stretch, 126, *126*
Tyson, Mike, xi
  decline of style/sloppiness, 28
  on fear, 8
  fights, 28, 55
  footwork, 28
  and jab, 12
  and power punches, 19

U

Uppercut, 17-18, *18*, 165
  right, 76, *77*
Us3, 59

V

V body shape, pull-ups for, 19
Visualization, xii
  for jab, 10, 73
V-sits, 124, *124*
  lateral, 125, *125*
V slip, 23, *23*
  and counters, 78

W

Waist exercises
  pivot jumps, 83, *83*
  torso twists, 63-64, *63, 64*
Warm-down. *See also* Cool-down
  stretching, 44
Warm-up. *See also* specific exercises
  advanced, 106-8
  beginners, 62-71
  professional fighters and, 44
  slow punching, 43
  stretching, 43
Weight-lifting, 19, 145
Women and Aerobox, xii, 144-45
  adolescent, 147
  and aggression, 144
  bladder/transient incontinence problems, 146
  bone health/osteoporosis prevention, 145
  clothing for workout/sports bra, 146
  menstruation, 147
  positive self-image, 146, *146*
  pregnancy, 147
  tricep toning (for flabby upper arms), 10

Y

Yoga stretch, 104, *104*

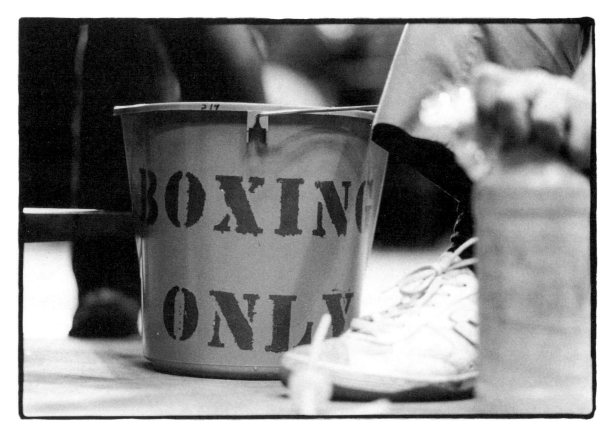

ANDREW BRUCKER